# Contents

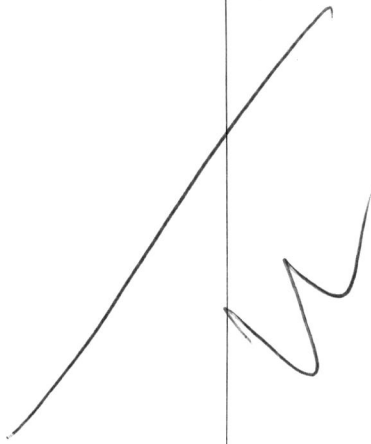

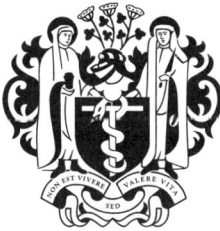

*The* ROYAL
SOCIETY *of*
MEDICINE
PRESS *Limited*

British Library Cataloguing in Publication Data

A catalogue record for this book is available from the British Library

ISBN 1–85315–473–3

Typeset by BA & GM Haddock, Woodlands, Ford, Midlthian EH37 5RE

Printed in Great Britain by Bell & Bain, Glasgow

# Preface

A recent survey of Internet usage amongst members' of the Royal Society of Medicine (RSM) highlighted the perennial problem many health professionals face when using the Internet - namely how difficult and time consuming it is to find high quality, information-rich Web sites. Too often a search of the Internet will direct the user to Web pages where the information is inaccurate, biased, out-of date, and irrelevant. Indeed, in the RSM survey around one third of all respondents commented that Internet searches typically identified 'too many irrelevant results', whilst around 20% of those surveyed confessed to be 'unable to find what they wanted'[1].

This book attempts to mitigate such problems by providing busy health professionals with a quick guide to be the best sources of health information on the Internet. Authored by recognised subject experts, each chapter provides a snapshot of the key resources that are available. Unless explicitly stated, all the resources described in this book are available free of charge.

The subjects selected for analysis include evidence based health care, health statistics and the increasingly important topic of genomics, whilst the more audience-focused pieces highlight the best Web sources for specialists such as obstetricians, orthopaedic surgeons and clinicians working in renal medicine. As no single book can hope to cover all areas of interest the final chapter provides the reader with a practical guide to how to the search the Web.

Originally published in *He@lth Information on the Internet*, these articles have all been revised and updated for this new publication. This book also has a supporting Web site <http://www.rsm.ac.uk/pub/bkkiley2.htm> that contains hypertext links to all the sites discussed herein. Through this site you can also mail me with any suggestions you have for subjects you would like covered in any future edition.

**Robert Kiley – Editor**
*Head of Systems Strategy*
*Wellcome Library for the History & Understanding of Medicine*

### Reference

1. Survey of RSM members' Internet use. Royal Society of Medicine, 2000. Results available online at: <http://www.rsm.ac.uk/new/websurvey.htm>

# 1

# Renal medicine on
# the Internet

Alastair J. Hutchison

*Manchester Institute of Nephrology and Transplantation*

ahutchison@renal.cmht.nwest.nhs.uk

## Introduction

Progressive renal disease leading to dialysis and kidney transplantation is relatively uncommon in comparison to other conditions such as ischaemic heart disease or cancer. Only around 90 to 110 new patients per million population in the UK require renal replacement therapy each year. Consequently, when a patient is told that they have 'kidney failure' they are likely to have great difficulty in acquiring further information about their diagnosis and prognosis.

Exposure to renal medicine at medical school has in the past been relatively poor, so that even the patient's general practitioner may have difficulty offering informed advice and counselling. In addition, the patient may never have met anyone else with a similar diagnosis, thereby increasing the feeling of loneliness and isolation. Paradoxically, successful management of renal replacement therapy requires a higher level of patient understanding and participation than almost any other condition with the exception, perhaps, of diabetes.

As recently as 1980, dialysis and kidney transplantation were only available to a minority of patients with end-stage renal disease, and information about renal disease was only to be found in a small number of specialist publications. The introduction of continuous ambulatory peritoneal dialysis allowed many more patients access to treatment and, in recent years, the Internet has made a wealth of information available to patients and healthcare professionals alike.

For patients with uncommon causes of kidney disease, the Internet provides a means of tracking down current research and practice that may result in them being more 'informed' than the professionals looking after them. Under these circumstances, medical staff need to catch up quickly, and be able to help the patient assess critically the validity of the information they obtain. In this way, the relationship with the patient can be greatly strengthened rather than weakened. Therefore, a working knowledge of what is available on the Internet within your own area of practice is essential.

## Starting points

There are perhaps four key sites for anyone in the UK wanting to find out more about renal disease, namely:

- **Nephronline** <http://www.nephronline.org/> – a new, commercially sponsored site for healthcare professionals involved in the management of patients with kidney disease, but which also contains a section specifically for patients and their carers.

- **National Kidney Federation** <http://www.kidney.org.uk/> – a site 'run by patients for patients'.

- **Hypertension, Dialysis and Clinical Nephrology (HDCN)** <http://www.hdcn.com/> – a site developed by the American Society of Nephrology in association with the Renal Physicians Association. Useful resources available here include recordings of presentations from major meetings, which are accompanied by online slides that appear automatically on your screen as you listen. Though access to all the information on this site incurs a registration fee of $65, it is perhaps the single most useful nephrological Web site available to renal professionals at present.

- **Sites on nephrology** <http://www.milach.com/complete.htm> – perhaps the most complete set of nephrology 'links' available on the Internet.

Not only are these sites each well constructed and informative, but the links provided within them give access to almost all the available, worthwhile nephrology sites – you almost need read no further! For readers who are interested in learning more about renal information on the Web, I will categorise additional useful renal sites under the following headings:

- Sites for renal professionals
- Sites that cover renal education and teaching
- Sites for patients and their carers

## Sites for renal professionals

### Professional associations

Despite renal medicine being a relatively small specialty, there is a multitude of professional societies and organisations, some of which only focus on a particular aspect of renal disease. This reflects the fact that renal failure can result from a wide variety of disease processes and, once established, can affect a wide variety of body systems. However, links to almost all these organisations can be found at the HDCN site (see above). The major European and US renal 'umbrella' societies all have good Web sites which provide a variety of services, including on-line registration for their annual meetings.

The British Renal Association's site <http://www.renal.org/index.htm> gives access to two particularly useful facilities – the Association's Standards Document, and a link to the UK Renal Registry at <http://www.renalreg.com/>. The Standards Document sets out the agreed guidelines and standards for management of patients with renal failure in the UK, whilst the Registry provides data on the extent to which these standards are being achieved (Fig. 1.1). The European Dialysis and Transplantation site <http://ftpwww.cce.unipr.it/%7Eeraedta/> is somewhat disappointing, but does provide a very useful password-protected database of the names, addresses and e-mail addresses of all its members.

Looking across the Atlantic, the sister organisation to the British Renal Association is the American Society of Nephrology <http://www.asn-online.com/>. Surprisingly, it is relatively limited in scope and belies the size and power of the Society, which organises the biggest annual renal meeting in the world.

Of much more interest is the United States Renal Data System (USRDS) <http://www.usrds.org/>, the US equivalent of the UK Renal Registry. The USRDS

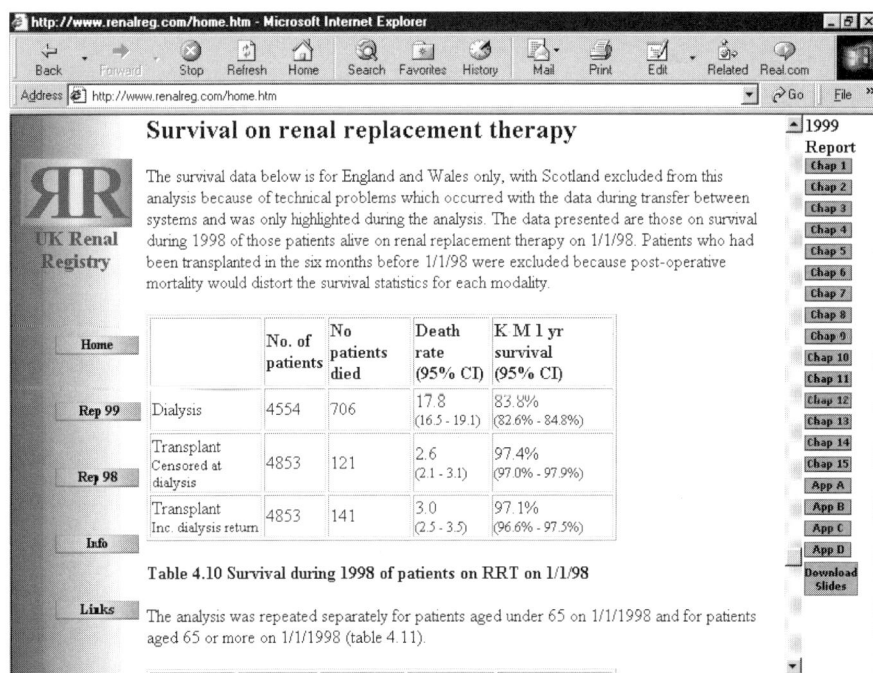

**Survival on renal replacement therapy**

The survival data below is for England and Wales only, with Scotland excluded from this analysis because of technical problems which occurred with the data during transfer between systems and was only highlighted during the analysis. The data presented are those on survival during 1998 of those patients alive on renal replacement therapy on 1/1/98. Patients who had been transplanted in the six months before 1/1/98 were excluded because post-operative mortality would distort the survival statistics for each modality.

| | No. of patients | No patients died | Death rate (95% CI) | K M 1 yr survival (95% CI) |
|---|---|---|---|---|
| Dialysis | 4554 | 706 | 17.8 (16.5 - 19.1) | 83.8% (82.6% - 84.8%) |
| Transplant Censored at dialysis | 4853 | 121 | 2.6 (2.1 - 3.1) | 97.4% (97.0% - 97.9%) |
| Transplant Inc. dialysis return | 4853 | 141 | 3.0 (2.5 - 3.5) | 97.1% (96.6% - 97.5%) |

Table 4.10 Survival during 1998 of patients on RRT on 1/1/98

The analysis was repeated separately for patients aged under 65 on 1/1/1998 and for patients aged 65 or more on 1/1/1998 (table 4.11).

**Fig. 1.1** Detailed and authoratitive data from the UK Renal Registry

collects, analyzes, and distributes information about end-stage renal disease in the US. The USRDS is the authoritative source of information on the demography of renal disease in the US, and it produces an annual report compiled from returns made by every US renal unit. The full text and graphics of the report are available online and, in addition, one can download a complete set of all the graphs and charts as a series of PowerPoint slides. E-mail requests can be made for data not available in the Annual Data Reports. Unlike the UK Renal Registry its data are purely demographic and it does not provide any information on achievement of standards.

US management standards for dialysis patients have recently been set by the National Kidney Foundation <http://www.kidney.org/>. The Kidney Disease Outcomes Quality Initiative guidelines <http://www.kidney.org/professionals/doqi/index.cfm> currently provide clinical management guidelines in four main areas of renal medicine – haemodialysis, peritoneal dialysis, vascular access and anaemia management.

Moving world-wide, the International Society of Nephrology has a US-based site <http://www.isn-online.org/> with a European mirror site <http://www. his.path.cam.ac.uk/mirrors/isn> in Cambridge, UK. Again, the site provides largely general information about the society with a link to its journal, *Kidney International*.

Examples of sub-specialty sites include the International Society of Renal Nutrition and Metabolism <http://wdsroot.ucdavis.edu/clients/renalsoc/default.html> and the excellent International Society for Peritoneal Dialysis site <http://www.ispd.org/>. This site contains a useful set of guidelines relevant to the management of peritoneal dialysis patients and an atlas of nearly 300 diagrams and microscopy slides relating to the peritoneum. It also links to its journal, *Peritoneal Dialysis International* at <http://www. multi-med.com/pdi/>.

## Disease-specific sites

Several disease-specific Web sites exist, usually dealing with relatively rare conditions. These are particularly useful because it is often difficult to find relevant, up to date information within conventional textbooks. A small list of links to such sites is provided by HDCN. Examples of conditions that even nephrologists have to look up from time to time are cystinosis and Fabry's syndrome. Cystinosis is a rare condition affecting only 1 in every 200,000 live births but several Web sites cover it, the best being Cystinosis Central <http://medicine.ucsd.edu/cystinosis/Index.htm> run by the Department of Pediatrics, University of California in San Diego. Fabry's syndrome is less rare (1 in 40,000), but again not well covered in the texts on my bookshelf. However, the Department of Human Genetics at Mount Sinai School of Medicine in New York describes it well on their Web site at <http://www. mssm.edu/crc/Fabry/fabry.html>. Since Fabry's syndrome has multi-system effects, another useful page of information is available from the National

Institute of Neurological Disorders and Stroke at <http://www.ninds.nih.gov/health_and_medical/disorders/fabrys_doc.htm>. Other rare conditions of all types may be looked up at the National Organisation for Rare Diseases site – <http://www.rarediseases.org/welcome.htm>

## Online Journals

Many medical journals of all descriptions are now available on-line, and although at one time it appeared that more and more were beginning to make their full content available to all, there is now a move towards subscription-only availability.

Nevertheless, all the major renal journals have a Web presence now, and one that deserves particular mention is the *American Journal of Kidney Diseases* – <http://www.ajkd.org/> published by NKF. This journal has used Web technology to speed up its peer review process. Reviewers can submit their critique of a submitted manuscript on-line, and the author can see at a glance how far through the process the article has gone. Confidentiality is maintained by the use of a unique manuscript number, known only to the author and the reviewers. Full text articles are only available to subscribers, as is the case with *Nephrology Dialysis Transplantation* <http://www.oup.co.uk/ndt/> and *Kidney International* <http://www.blackwell-synergy.com/issuelist.asp?journal=kid>.

## Drug information

One of the common problems that non-nephrologists have in dealing with renal patients is drug dosages. The British National Formulary <http://bnf.org/> contains an appendix on prescribing in renal disease, whilst a privately run site provides a variety of useful information and online calculators at <http://home.eznet.net/~webtent/renalpharmacology.html>.

# Sites for renal education and teaching

Renal pathology is a confusing subject and textbooks that cover this are inevitably expensive because of the small number of sales. However, several good sites provide both case histories and high quality renal histology images. The Virtual Hospital from the University of Iowa has a clear explanation of glomerulonephritis at <http://www.vh.org/Providers/Textbooks/GN/GNHP.html>. Clinico-pathological cases are also available from Harvard University, <http://www.isn-online.org/start.htm> courtesy of the ISN. The ISN Web site also provides access to the Atlas of Diseases of the Kidney at <http://www. kidneyatlas.org/> (Fig. 1.2). This comprehensive five volume textbook with over 2500 images covers all areas of nephrology. Full text searching is supported as is the downloading of full screen colour images.

Surprisingly, one of the most comprehensive educational sites is provided by the US Army Medical Center Nephrology Service at <http://www.wramc.amedd.army.mil/departments/medicine/nephrology/>. This sites contains over 30 PowerPoint

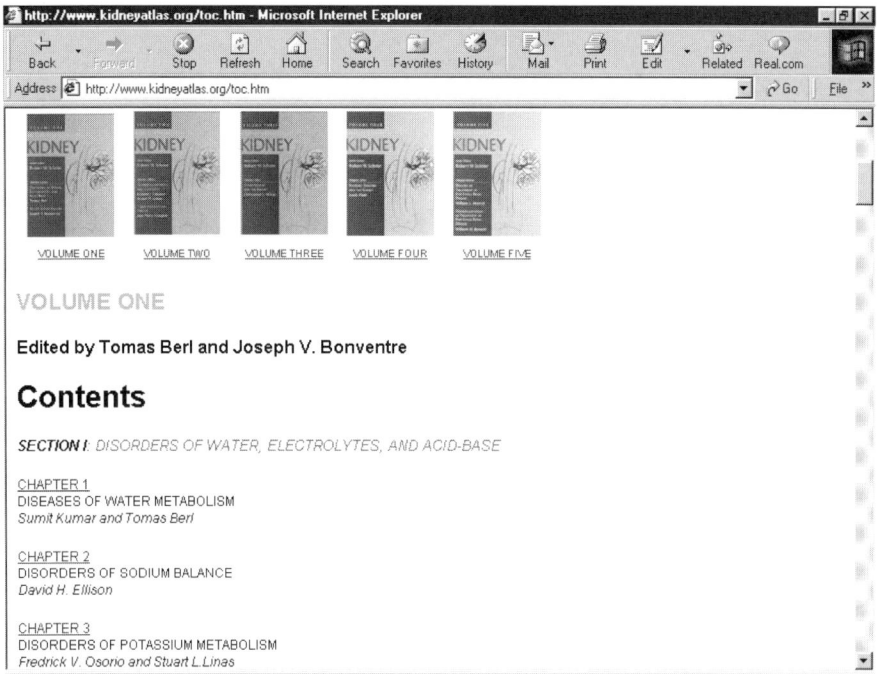

**Fig. 1.2** Kidney Atlas – over 2500 online images

presentations on a variety of renal topics, all of which are down-loadable. Some of the presentations also have a follow-up quiz attached. Although these slides could be used for self-directed learning they would be better used by an expert as part of a lecture. The US Army site also has a set of useful calculators, one of which allows entry of serum creatinines from a patient with progressive renal impairment, and then produces a graphical plot to estimate the date at which dialysis will probably become necessary. The programme can be downloaded as an Excel file and with small modifications will work with SI units rather than mg/dl. This is a useful tool which I use in clinical practise.

## Sites for patients and their carers

Many of the sites discussed above have sections for patients and carers, but there are three particularly good starting points. The UK National Kidney Federation <http://www.kidney.org.uk/> runs an excellent site, with full and accurate information about the Federation as well as up to date news, recommended books, medical information and FAQs (Fig. 1.3). In addition it has useful links, and complete details of how to contact a local Kidney Patient Association indexed by town or local hospital. The site has a confident and reliable feel to it which is so important to an anxious patient.

The Kidney Patient Guide <http://www.kidneypatientguide.org.uk/site/ contents.html> is another useful site. This site is overseen by a nephrologist, Dr

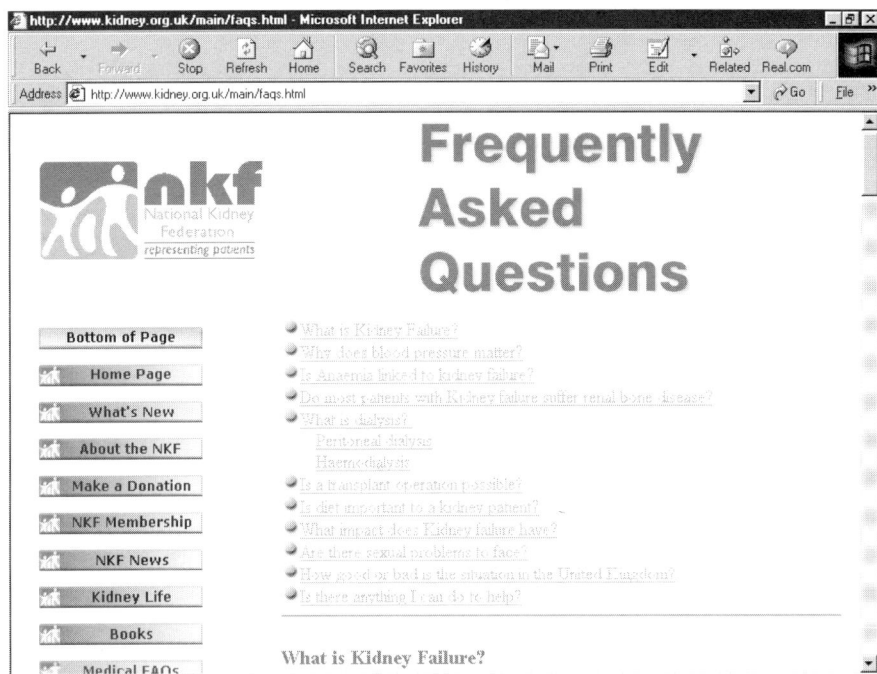

**Fig. 1.3** FAQs at the National Kidney Federation site

Peter Rutherford and is sponsored by a Wellcome Trust grant. In addition to a wealth of useful and accurate information, there is an online (and very active) bulletin board supervised by Dr Rutherford.

The UK NKF's American equivalent is a branch of the US National Kidney Foundation (which confusingly shares the same initials). This organisation is called the Patient and Family Council <http://www.kidney.org/patients/>. Its site takes a similar approach to its UK cousin but has a slightly less friendly feel to it. However, its 'A to Z guide' is a very useful source of detailed information even if at times some of the American terminology might be confusing.

## Conclusion

The World Wide Web provides professionals and patients with rapid access to information that would have been almost impossible to find only 10 years ago. It particularly excels in smaller specialty areas of medicine such as nephrology. Resources such as the National Organisation for Rare Diseases enable dissemination of information about conditions of which many physicians have little or no recollection. Patients with such conditions are obviously encountered infrequently, but are increasingly likely to have utilised the Internet to find current information before they enter the specialist's consulting room. This presents a new challenge to the 'doctor–patient relationship' for which one must be well prepared by being aware of available resources on the Internet.

# 2

# Sifting for evidence: a guide to EBHC on the Internet

Andrew Booth BA, MSc, DipLib, ALA

*Director of Information Resources and Senior Lecturer in Evidence Based Healthcare Information, School of Health and Related Research (ScHARR), University of Sheffield*

a.booth@sheffield.ac.uk

## Introduction

Evidence-based healthcare[1] (EBHC), a new paradigm aimed at stimulating the quality of clinical care through the utilisation of research findings, has spawned a minor industry of books, journals and CD-ROM products. The opportune timing of this new approach to coincide with the rapid development of the Internet has resulted in the World Wide Web (WWW) being harnessed as an alternative delivery mechanism or, at the very least, dual text-based and electronic publications. With access to the WWW becoming less of an issue, concern now centres on whether the Internet can be regarded as a reliable channel for the delivery of relevant, timely and accurate patient-focused information. How practical is it for a busy healthcare worker to use the Web in sifting for 'evidence'?

In an article in the first-ever issue of *He@lth Information on the Internet* (February 1998)[2] this author demonstrated that it was indeed feasible for a healthcare worker to attempt to locate answers to clinical scenarios. In fairness, however, the approaches presented there were comparatively unstructured, especially alongside the precision previously afforded by bibliographic databases such as MEDLINE with its Medical Subject Headings (MeSH) vocabulary and its pre-defined content and scope. For an approach to be successful required a comprehensive knowledge of evidence based sources, the ability to recognise a high-quality source from a brief perusal of a result summary, and expertise in identifying the characteristics of particular question types.

11

The intervening years have seen great improvements for the less-experienced evidence-seeker, particularly with the development of a number of one-stop gateways or evidence filters. Such is their utility that they have become the 'first resort' for almost any clinically based evidence scenario. The three leading resources, prominently placed on my personal toolbar, are:

1. Turning Research Into Practice (TRIP) Database <http://www.tripdatabase.com>.
   A meta-resource indexing the contents of 26 different high-quality evidence sources comprising over 10,000 individual links.

2. PubMed Medline Clinical Filters page <http://www.ncbi.nlm.nih.gov/entrez/query/static/clinical.html>.
   This interface to the National Library of Medicine's MEDLINE database restricts subject searches to high-quality articles by looking for methodological terms (e.g. 'randomized controlled trial') in the title, abstract or index (MeSH) terms.

3. SUMSearch <http://sumsearch.uthscsa.edu/searchform45.htm>.
   This search interface, developed by the Society for General Internal Medicine, runs a subject query against a number of high quality resources such as filtered MEDLINE, the NHS Centre for Reviews and Dissemination's Database of Abstracts of Reviews of Effectiveness (DARE) and the National Guideline Clearinghouse (U.S.).

In addition to the potential of improved technical facilities as described above, there is also a greater awareness of how techniques developed elsewhere for evidence-based information retrieval can be applied to searching for evidence on the Internet. These techniques include:

1. Focusing the question using the 'PICO' anatomy <http://www.shef.ac.uk/~scharr/ir/focusing.html>. This is done by deconstructing any clinical query into the four elements of the Patient or Problem, the Intervention of interest, the Comparison intervention and the intended Outcomes. This improves the precision of the search query.

2. Filtering results using methodological terms <http://www.shef.ac.uk/~scharr/ir/filter.html>. This is done by qualifying a subject query with terms likely to occur in higher quality articles. This improves the validity of the search results.

This chapter revisits the three scenarios used in the previous article not only to identify new subject resources that may have appeared over the last three years but also, more importantly, to utilise the new technical facilities and techniques outlined above. In this way I hope to demonstrate the potential that the Internet – the infrastructure that underpins the NHSNet – may yet realise to the benefit of healthcare workers, researchers and patients.

***Scenario 1:*** *The drug information officer at a local NHS Trust seeks information on the use of low molecular weight heparin (LWMH) for the treatment of deep vein thrombosis (DVT). What evidence is available on the World Wide Web?*

Using the focused question technique we identify the Problem as 'deep vein thrombosis' and the Intervention as 'low molecular weight heparin'. The Comparison and Outcomes are unspecified but could be added subsequently, if required.

The TRIP database is a comparatively small collection of electronic records and simple search terms (words or phrases) can be used because a searcher will usually be prepared to 'eyeball' the initial search results. Because the TRIP database only indexes the <u>titles</u> of the records we decide to employ two separate search strategies — the first a 'Problem' search for 'deep vein thrombosis' (remembering to return to the search screen to try 'DVT' and 'deep venous thrombosis' as follow-up alternatives) and the second using the 'Intervention' search 'heparin'. (Fig. 2.1)

The impressive result-sets list titles as hypertext links to resources such as the Cochrane Abstracts <u><http://www.update-software.com/cochrane/cochrane-frame.html></u>[3], the ACP Journal Club <u><http://www.acponline.org/></u>[4] and DARE <u><http://agatha.york.ac.uk/welcome.htm></u> as well as to critically appraised summaries such

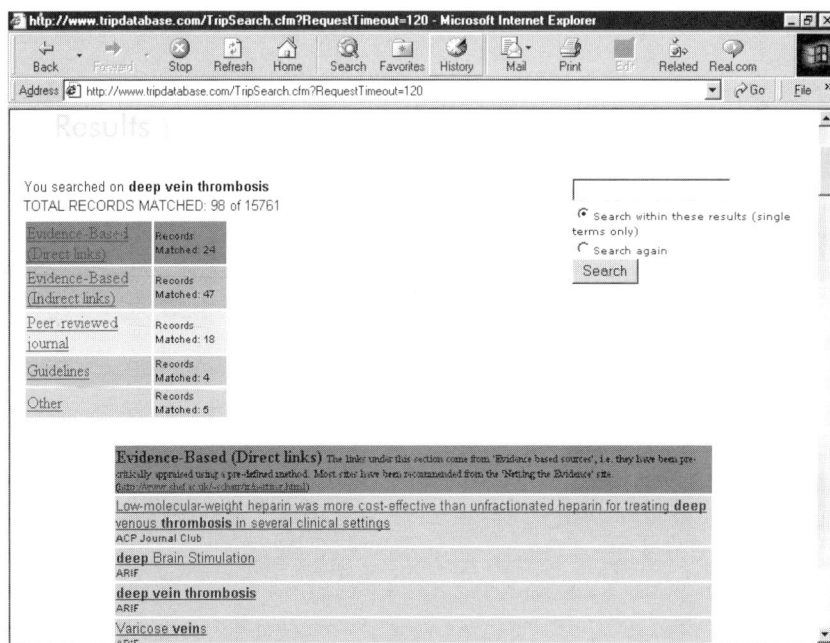

Fig. 2.1  A TRIP database search on 'deep vein thrombosis'.

as Journal Club on the Web <http://www.journalclub.org> and the *Journal of Family Practice* Problem Oriented Evidence that Matters (POEMS) <http://www.infopoems.com/POEMs/POEMs Home.htm>. There is also a Web page, although quite dated, reporting the result of an information request submitted to the Aggressive Research Intelligence Facility (ARIF) in the West Midlands <http://www.hsrc.org.uk/links/arif/deep.htm> that references two systematic reviews together with accompanying commentary.

When moving on to use the PubMed Clinical Queries option we decide to be more precise in our searching as our search will run across 11 million-plus records from the MEDLINE database. We therefore type in our Problem (deep vein thrombosis) and our Intervention (in full – low molecular weight heparin). These terms will be combined by the MEDLINE interface so that we will only retrieve records that contain both the problem and the intervention. We then specify our question type by checking the option marked 'therapy' – this will activate a filter that looks predominantly for clinical trials. Other options include diagnosis, prognosis and aetiology. Finally, we decide whether we want the filter to be applied sensitively (to retrieve more records at the possible cost of quality) or specifically (to retrieve fewer records but of higher quality). The search is then run using these parameters. A valuable feature of PubMed is the flag marked 'Related' which is placed beside each search result. This allows us to click on a relevant record and thus automatically run a search using that record's key words.

Finally, the SUMSearch facility combines features from both TRIP and PubMed in that it runs filters against MEDLINE, again activated by checking a box against the relevant question type, but supplements results from acknowledged high quality resources such as DARE and the National Guidelines Clearinghouse. SUMSearch has the same filters as PubMed (i.e. therapy, diagnosis, prognosis and causation) but augmented by physical findings and screening. We focus our question in the suggested manner so as to retrieve only those records containing 'deep vein thrombosis' and 'low molecular weight heparin' and dealing with therapy questions.

The extent of our results for this search probably eliminates any need to broaden our search to more general search engines. It is increasingly recognised that even the best of these search engines indexes less than a third of the indexable Web. Had our retrieval results been poor using the three specialist engines we could have proceeded to AltaVista Advanced Queries option which would allow us to enter a precise Problem-Intervention query ('low molecular weight heparin' AND 'deep vein thrombosis'). However, the recent availability of the tool Copernic2000 <http://www.copernic.com>, a search engine that allows searching of multiple search engines and the filtering and storage of results, means that we can search for any page that has all our chosen search words specifying anywhere between 100 (Quick Search) and 1000 (Custom) results. As Copernic2000 is run from our local PC we can download all the relevant pages and sift through them offline.

**Scenario 2:** *A junior doctor has been following the debate about the use of beta interferon for multiple sclerosis and wants to identify evidence on its effectiveness and cost-effectiveness.*

New drugs, and to a lesser extent other new technologies, suggest that likely sources of evidence will include health technology assessment (HTA) agencies and their prodigious output of assessment reports. Fortunately resources covered by TRIP include the NHS Centre for Reviews and Dissemination's (NHSCRD) Health Technology Assessment database <http://agatha.york.ac.uk/welcome.htm> and the full-text reports produced under the NHS HTA Programme <http://www.hta.nhsweb.nhs.uk/htapubs.htm> Such reports often cover cost effectiveness issues as well as those around clinical effectiveness. Technology assessment is typically conducted at both a national and a regional level so other useful resources will include the regional HTA reports produced by South and West Development and Evaluation Committee <http://www.hta.nhsweb.nhs.uk/rapidhta/html_summaries/77.htm>, West Midlands Development and Evaluation Service <http://web.bham.ac.uk/stewaray/> and the Trent Working Group on Acute Purchasing <http://www.shef.ac.uk/uni/academic/R-Z/tiwgap/>. Our search of TRIP yields some of the resources that appeared for the previous query such as ACP Journal Club and the Abstracts of Cochrane Reviews, as well as additional resources such as the Centre for Evidence Based Medicine's Critically Appraised Topics (CAT) Bank <http://cebm.jr2.ox.ac.uk/cats/ms_beta-interferon.html>. CATs are one page patient-specific summaries that summarise rigorous research evidence and then disseminate the findings using tailored software called CAT-Maker.

For specific coverage of cost-effectiveness issues the recommended resource is another NHSCRD database, the NHS Economic Evaluations Database (NEED) <http://agatha.york.ac.uk/welcome.htm>. This database consists of economic studies identified from MEDLINE and other databases but enhanced by the addition of value-added structured abstracts compiled by health economists.

Interferon can be used to treat many conditions so specificity is added to our search by using the precise form of interferon (interferon beta) in conjunction with the specific Problem (multiple sclerosis). If we were particularly interested in a specific Outcome then a search using our meta-search engine Copernic2000 would be modified by adding outcome-related words such as 'relapse'. Our Copernic2000 search yields the report of an NHS HTA Programme project <http://www.hta.nhsweb.nhs.uk/projdets/950102.htm> and a technology overview from the Canadian Coordinating Office for Health Technology Assessment <http://www.ccohta.ca/pubs/beta_1b-e.html>.

*Scenario 3 :* A multidisciplinary group led by nurses and physiotherapists wishes to develop guidelines on the treatment of back pain. Is there any evidence on the Web?

Up until recent years there was no 'one-stop' resource for guidelines. However, the appearance of the National Guideline Clearinghouse <http://www.guidelines.gov/> (U.S.) has improved the situation (Fig. 2.2). If you are specifically looking for guidelines material, as opposed to high-quality evidence in general, then you should prioritise a direct visit to the National Guideline Clearinghouse site over use of the evidence portals mentioned above. TRIP does include coverage of other guideline sources such as the Canadian Medical Association's Clinical Practice Guidelines Infobase <http://www.cma.ca/cpgs/index.asp> but the PubMed and SUMSearch interfaces have little to offer for guidelines over and above a conventional MEDLINE search using 'guideline' or 'practice guideline' as the publication type limiter.

The National Guideline Clearinghouse site allows such features as comparing structured evaluations of two or more guidelines and has links to full-text where available. From the Clearinghouse the aforementioned enquirers would be able to read full-text statements such as the AHCPR's *Acute low back problems in adults: assessment and treatment* and the US Preventative Services Task Force's

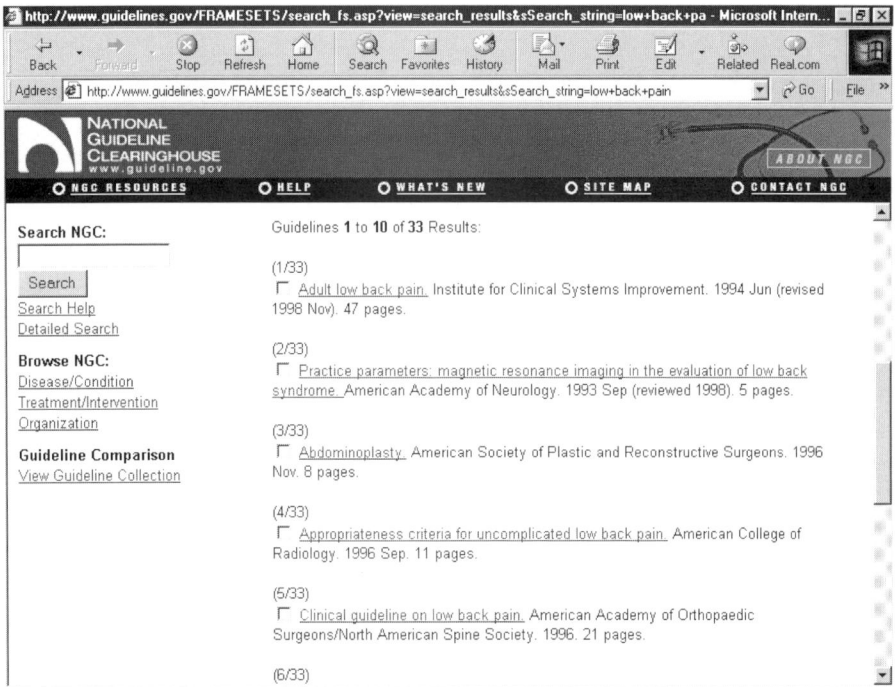

**Fig. 2.2** The National Guideline Clearinghouse (US) Web site.

*Counseling to prevent low back pain.* Of course, in the absence of such published guidelines you might choose to return to the PubMed Clinical Queries interface for original clinical trials covering diagnosis or treatment of the condition in question.

When using the National Guideline Clearinghouse site caution must be exercised because of its US bias. A guideline search of this resource will usually need to be supplemented by a search using a general search engine, preferably a meta-search engine such as Copernic2000. It is in using a general search engine to find a specific publication type, such as a guideline, that the principle of filtering mentioned earlier comes into its own. Here you conduct a subject search, perhaps focused on the 'Problem' component of a focused question e.g. 'low back pain', and then add a suitable filter term such as 'guideline' or 'practice parameter' or 'clinical pathway'. This restricts retrieval to only those documents that contain the filter <u>and</u> the subject terms.

You should note that when using a general search engine a clinical term such as 'low back pain' should be preferred to the less specific 'back pain' as it is more likely that retrieved documents will be clinically-focused. The technique of limiting to a specific publication type works in the same way for therapy questions using terms such as 'clinical trial', 'controlled trial' or 'randomised trial' and for general systematic review-type questions using 'systematic review', 'meta-analysis' or 'overview'. Our general search using Copernic2000 with our guidelines filter retrieves such useful documents as the Royal College of General Practitioners' National Low Back Pain Clinical Guidelines <http://www.rcgp.org.uk/rcgp/clinspec/guidelines/backpain/> the New Zealand Guidelines Group's Acute Low Back Pain Guide <http://www.nzgg.org.nz/library/gl_complete/backpain1/full_text.cfm> and the New South Wales Therapeutic Assessment Group's Low Back Pain Guidelines for GPs <http://www.medeserv.com.au/tag/guidelines/lbp_gp1.htm>

## Conclusion

Although the volume of clinically relevant materials on the Internet has grown exponentially over the last few years it is still true to say that there are three main types of evidence-based information product – the critically appraised topic, the health technology assessment report and the clinical guideline. The development of evidence portals over recent years has made the identification of previously isolated pockets of evidence much easier. At the same time information management techniques, such as focusing the question and use of filters, have made sifting the evidence much more efficient.

The 'evidence seeker' wishing to become familiar with the landmarks of Evidence Based Practice, in contrast to the topic-based approach explored here, should start instead from a comprehensive resource list such as the author's own

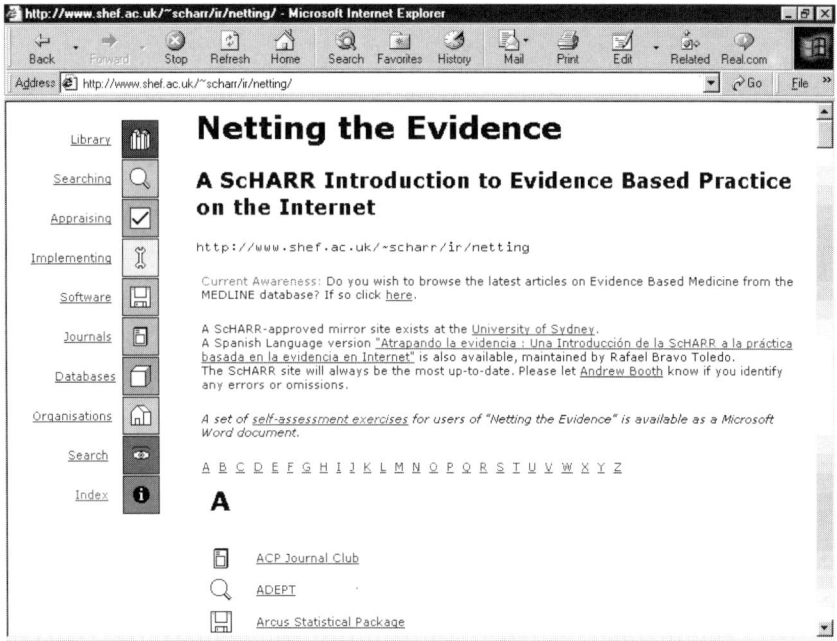

**Fig. 2.3** ScHARR *Netting the Evidence*

'Netting the Evidence' <http://www.shef.ac.uk/~scharr/ir/netting/> (Fig. 2.3). In addition to the source materials of evidence-based healthcare, enthusiasts will find links to software tools, toolkits, teaching materials and organisations to support their quest. May the evidence be with you!

## References

1. Muir Gray J A (1996) *Evidence-based health care: how to make health policy and management decisions*. London: Churchill Livingstone
2. Booth A. Following the evidence trail: EBHC on the Internet. *Health Information on the Internet* 1998; 1: 4–5 <http://www.wellcome.ac.uk/en/1/homlibinfacthiiarc1fol.html> [Accessed 7 September 2000]
3. Heparin, low molecular weight heparin and physical methods for preventing deep vein thrombosis and pulmonary embolism following surgery for hip fractures <http://www.update-software.com/ccweb/cochrane/revabstr/ab000305.htm> [Accessed 7 September 2000]
4. Low-molecular-weight heparin was more cost-effective than unfractionated heparin for treating deep venous thrombosis in several clinical settings <http://www.acponline.org/journals/acpjc/marapr99/heparin.htm> [Accessed 7 September 2000]

# 3

# Mental health information on the Internet

## Andre Tomlin

*Director of Knowledge Services, Centre for Evidence-Based Mental Health,*
*University of Oxford, UK*

andre.tomlin@psych.ox.ac.uk

## Introduction

Mental health professionals suffer from the same problem of information overload as all other health professionals, and getting connected to the Internet only confounds this problem. Web surfers soon realise that there is more information available over the Internet than they ever dreamt possible, and the majority of it is not presented in a user-friendly or digestible way. So, like all other specialties, mental health sites need to organise their resources in a way that is more focused to the needs of the audience. They must also be constantly appraising and excluding the poor quality sites that make up the vast majority of the Web.

Some information professionals are beginning to develop gateways to high quality evidence, which can be used as a first port of call for a specific inquiry. These gateways are generally based on a similar model, the major health care examples being the National Electronic Library for Health (NeLH) <http://www.nelh.nhs.uk> and OMNI <http://omni.ac.uk>. Using a resource such as OMNI can help to alleviate the sensation of aimless drifting that all Web users have experienced at one time or another, as it provides fast access to high quality resources. At present there is not a mental health version of OMNI on the Web, although OMNI does include a number of useful mental health sites. A more recent, and altogether more comprehensive development is the National Electronic Library for Mental Health (NeLMH) <http://www.nelmh.org> (Fig. 3.1), a virtual branch library within the main NeLH that will offer fast access to

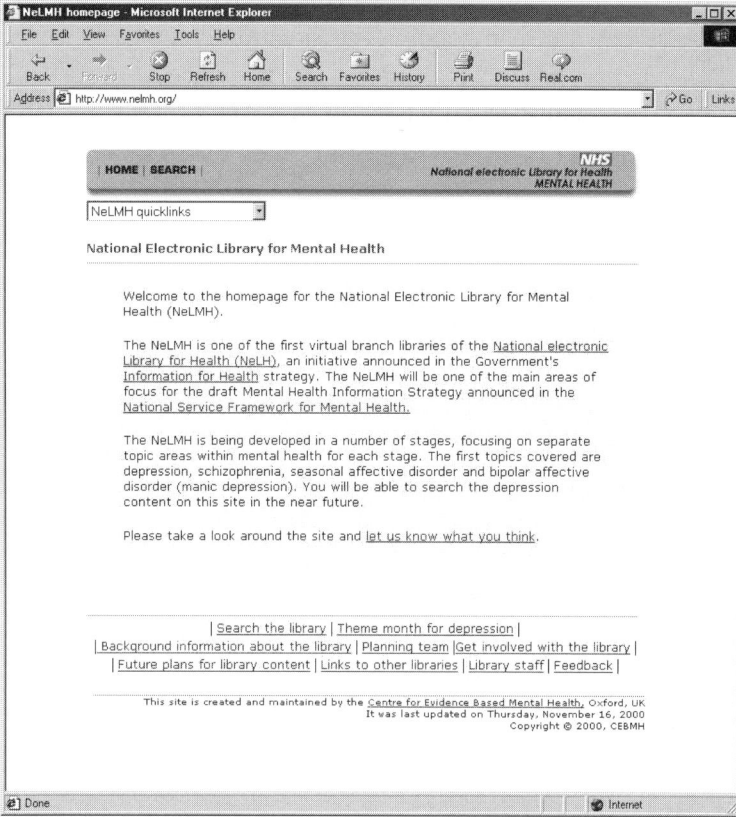

**Fig. 3.1** The National Electronic Library for Mental Health (NeLMH) Web site.

mental health knowledge for a wide variety of users including patients and health professionals.

In this article, I will describe some of the important mental health resources available on the Internet, dividing the resources into four main areas:

(i) patient information;

(ii) major organisational resources;

(iii) continuing medical education resources; and

(iv) where to go to find answers to mental health questions.

## Patient information

General patient information is not difficult to find on the Internet. A simple AltaVista search on patient or consumer information on the Internet retrieves nearly 4 million pages. However, as recent articles have shown, not everything out there is relevant and useful. Indeed, a great deal of the information provided may be doing more harm than good[1,2]. This situation has helped to ensure the success of a number of Web sites that seek to eradicate the problem of misinformation. – a movement that is spearheaded by retired psychiatrist, Stephen Barrett and his Quackwatch <http://www.quackwatch.com> site.

So where can mental health patients go to find reliable information on the Web? Well, there are a number of Web organisations that seek to provide reliable and up-to-date information to patients and their relatives to help them find out more about their illness. Three sites worth mentioning are:

1  NHS Direct Online <http://www.nhsdirect.nhs.uk>. Though this site covers all aspects of health, there is a significant amount of value-added, evidence-based mental health information for patients and their carers, courtesy of the NeLMH theme-months initiative. Subjects covered so far include depression <http://cebmh.com/depression.html>, with plans for further subjects in the future (Fig. 3.2).

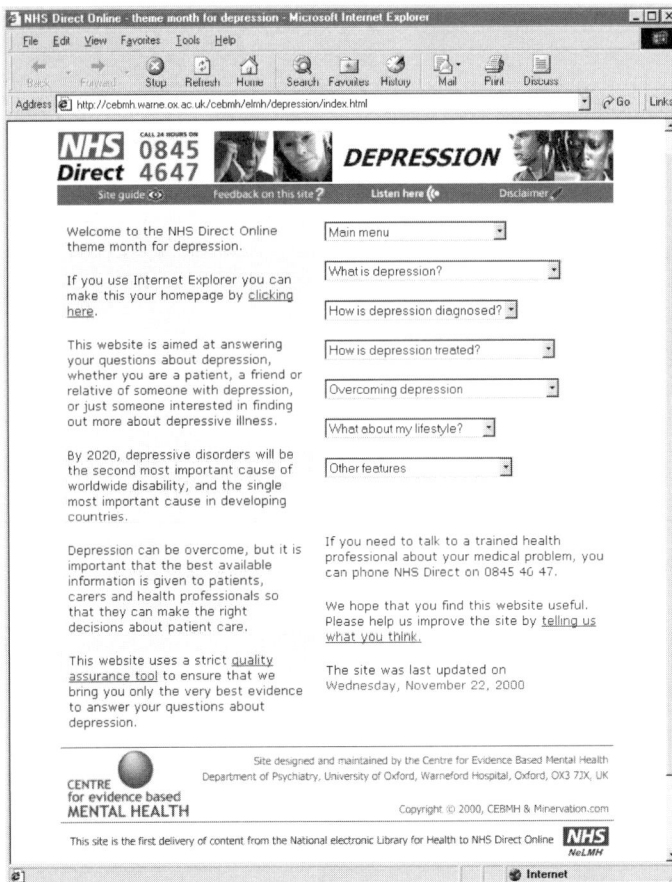

**Fig. 3.2** NHS Direct Online Depression <http://cebmh.com/depression.html> Web site

2   Internet Mental Health <http://www.mentalhealth.com>. Developed by Canadian psychiatrist Dr Philip Long, this site has detailed and well-structured information on the 54 most common mental disorders and the 72 most common psychiatric drugs. It also provides an interactive on-line tool as an aid to diagnosing various conditions such as anxiety disorders, mood disorders, schizophrenia and personality disorders.

3   Mental Help Net <http://mentalhelp.net/>. Sponsored by CHMC Systems, this site divides each mental health disorder into symptoms, treatment, resources, organisations and support.

In addition to these large resources, there are the smaller UK based sites provided by charities and government organisations. These range from the Mental Health Foundation <http://www.mentalhealth.org.uk> and the Sainsbury Centre for Mental Health <http://www.sainsburycentre.org.uk> to The Royal College of Psychiatrists <http://www.rcpsych.ac.uk/public/help/welcome.htm> *Help is at Hand* patient information leaflets.

## Major organisational resources

The majority of large mental health organisations world-wide now have some kind of Web presence. These sites offer a variety of resources, ranging from guidelines and audit protocols, to research funding and training initiatives. The quality of these resources is extremely variable, and it is clear that many organisations have not yet

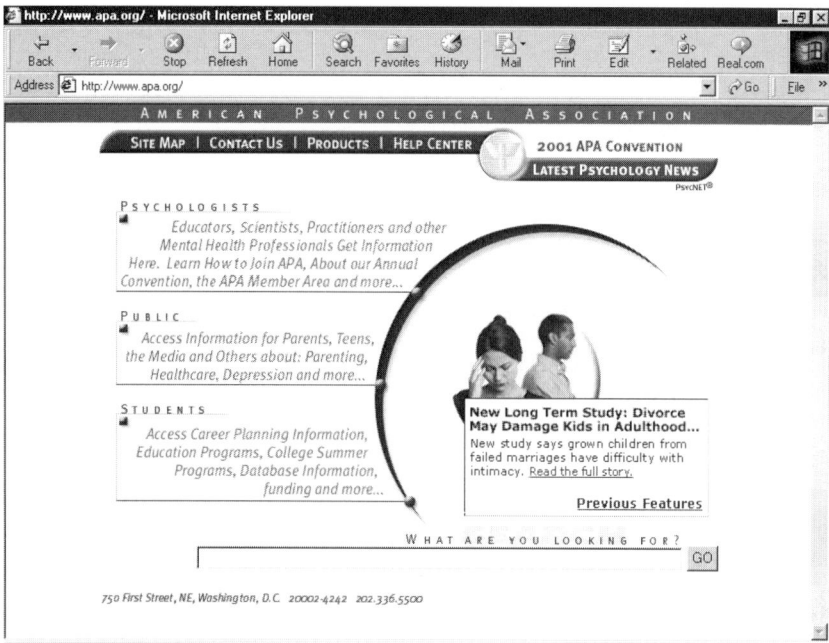

**Fig. 3.3** The American Psychological Association Web site.

reached the point where they are using their sites as a means for effective dissemination of information. However, sites worth visiting to get a flavour of what is available at present include the American Psychiatric Association <http://-www.psych.org>, the American Psychological Association <http://www.apa.org> (Fig. 3.3), the World Psychiatric Association <http://www.wpanet.org>, and in the UK The Royal College of Psychiatrists <http://www.rcpsych.ac.uk> and the British Psychological Society <http://www.bps.org.uk>.

Clinical practice guidelines relevant to mental health can also often be found on more general health care sites, and so users may also find it worthwhile visiting some of these. A good place to start a search such as this is the ScHARR guideline list <http://www.shef.ac.uk/~scharr/ir/guidelin.html>. The UK Royal College of Psychiatrists guidelines and evidence-based briefings are also available on the Web at <http://cebmh.warne.ox.ac.uk/cebmh/guidelines>.

## Continuing medical education resources

Web users searching for information on continuing medical education (CME) may find useful sections within the large organisational sites listed above. CME resources are generally not the first piece of information to be added to a Web site, and so the US based sites tend to have more detailed sections than their UK equivalents. Indeed the US has its own mental health CME site (complete with multimedia library) called the Mental Health Infosource <http://www.mhsource.com>. The US sites also currently lead the field in developing more innovative ways of providing continuing education, with sites such as audioPsych <http://www.audioPsych.com>, which uses a multimedia approach utilising RealAudio and interactive discussion forums.

General training resources are also available for mental health professionals over the Web, although they often form part of a larger Web site with no mental health focus. One site that does offer a tool kit of resources specifically aimed at implementing evidence-based practice in mental health is the Centre for Evidence Based Mental Health <http://cebmh.com>. This site offers a variety of tools to help users find, appraise and act upon evidence relating to their area of interest.

## Where to go to find answers to mental health questions?

So where are the really useful resources that give users exactly what they want within the 5 minute coffee break that they have allowed themselves to surf the Web? There is a handful of sites that offers access to critically appraised structured abstracts of systematic reviews and randomised controlled trials. These will always be the first port of call for questions of a therapeutic nature, and as they grow these sites will become increasingly important resources.

The three key resources in this group are:

1    The Cochrane Library <http://www.update-software.com/clibhome/clib.htm>. Abstracts can be read free of charge, though an annual fee of £120.00 is payable if you want access to the full database.

2    The journal *Evidence Based Mental Health* <http://www.ebmentalhealth.com>, published by BMJ Publishing.

3    *Clinical Evidence* <http://www.clinicalevidence.org>. This book, like the EBMH journal, contains a wide range of reliable abstracted information relevant to most areas of mental health.

The resource that brings all of these sources (and many more) together is the National Electronic Library for Mental Health (NeLMH) <http://www.nelmh.org>. This project started out as a UK National Health Service funded initiative, developing a virtual library of mental health knowledge for NHS professionals and patients. It has since grown to become a global project, aiming to develop a database that can be adapted to meet the needs of developing countries and US Health Maintenance Organizations (HMOs).

The electronic library is a comprehensive, reliable, unbiased and evidence based resource. In addition, it presents information to patients and their carers, mental health and primary care professionals, and health policy decision makers, in a format which they can quickly understand and digest. As it grows it will become the number one place to go if you have a question concerning a mental health issue.

### References

1   Bader SA, Braude RM. 'Patient informatics': creating new partnerships in medical decision making. *Acad Med* 1998; **73**: 408–11

2   McClung HJ, Murray RD, Heitlinger LA. The Internet as a source for current patient information. *Pediatrics* 1998; **101**: E2

# 4

# Health statistics on the Web

Julie Glanville

*Information Service Manager, Centre for Health Economics/NHS Centre for Reviews and Dissemination, University of York, York, UK*

jmg1@york.ac.uk

## Introduction

Statistics on disease, population, the healthcare process and health outcomes would seem to be ideal material for publication via the Web. Statistical information is usually highly structured, often in tables, and has table titles, rows and column headings which would seem to be ready made for retrieval by Web search engines. Paper versions of statistics are often problematic to use because they lack indexes and can involve much page scanning to find the information you seek.

However, though there is a growing volume of official and unofficial health statistics on the Web, the coverage is still not comprehensive and the provision of question-oriented search engines is poor. Indeed one key use of the Web currently seems to be as an index to what statistics have been published in paper form!

This brief paper is necessarily selective and presents some key UK sites along with suggestions about useful Internet guides, strategies for searching out statistical information and published guidance[1-3].

## Official statistics

The Department of Health (DoH) has taken a notable lead in this area and now routinely publishes many of its statistical publications on the Web. These can be accessed at <http://www.doh.gov.uk/public/stats1.htm> (Fig. 4.1). This is the site to visit for a wide range of health and health service statistics including waiting list

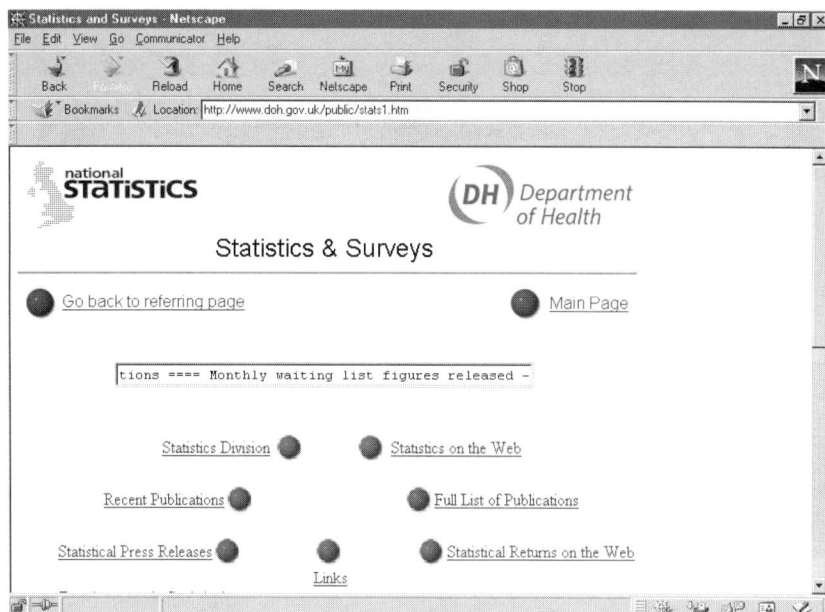

**Fig. 4.1** The UK Department of Health (DoH) statistical publications site.

figures, the Health Survey for England <http://www.doh.gov.uk/public/summary1.htm> and the National Survey of NHS patients <http://www.doh.gov.uk/public/gpn98tables.htm> as well as other surveys on health-related behaviour such as drinking, smoking and sun exposure. Tables from the annual Health and Personal Social Services Statistics (HPSSS) are provided in full and with a useful index <http://www.doh.gov.uk/HPSSS/INDEX.HTM>. The DoH site also provides Web access to the valuable Statistical Bulletins, which can be difficult to obtain in paper form. These report on health service manpower, health service usage and morbidity.

Routes into Scottish health statistics can be found via <http://www.scotland.gov.uk/stats/default.htm>, Northern Ireland statistics via <http://www.nisra.gov.uk/index.htm> and Welsh statistics at <http://www.wales.gov.uk/index_e.html>.

To find a way through the wealth of potentially useful statistics in order to answer a very specific question is, however, somewhat difficult. The DoH Web site offers the DoH search option that searches the whole Web site, not just statistics. This means that a simple search on 'angina' entered in the hope of finding out how many people are treated in the NHS for angina each year, produced 34 hits. From scanning those pages, the Health Survey for England statistics are found which report the percentage of people with angina and cardiovascular disease. Sifting through the 34 hits also produced some interesting background material.

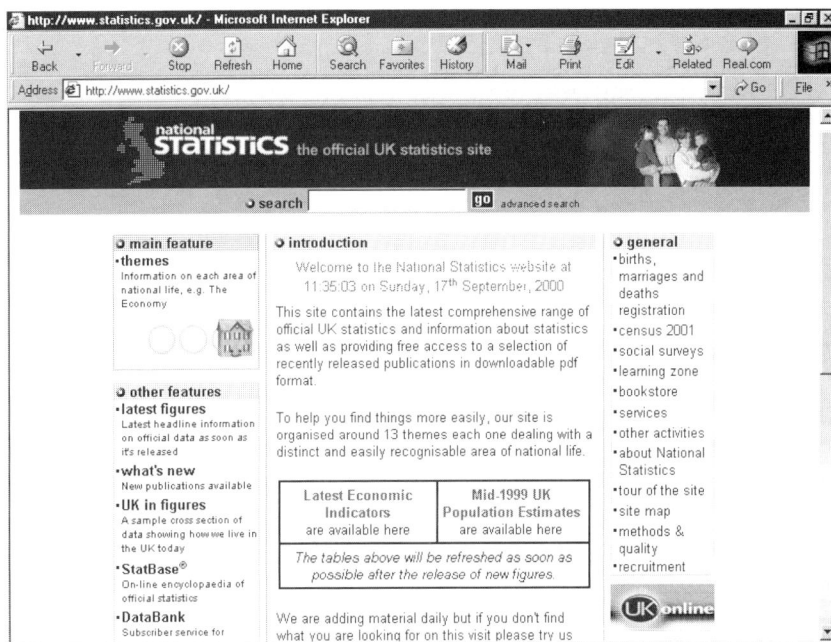

**Fig. 4.2** The UK Government Statistical Service.

The Government Statistical Service offers Web access to UK facts and figures at <http://www.statistics.gov.uk/> (Fig. 4.2). This is a gateway service to search-able collections such as Statbase, press releases and UK in Figures. There is, however, no overall search engine at this site that might provide a means to focus on optimal sites for specific questions.

Statbase <http://www.statistics.gov.uk/statbase/mainmenu.asp> provides access to official UK national statistics, many of which are accessible in full from this service. The datasets searched provide statistics on social trends, regional trends, health-related behaviour, waiting lists and cancer epidemiology. Using the text search facility on this site was unsuccessful for 'angina', but more successful when searching for 'heart disease'. A Statbase search produced statistics on premature deaths from circulatory diseases and cancers from Social Trends and also the prevalence of treated coronary heart disease and stroke. If a text search does not prove helpful, there is another search option – Statsearch. This presents the resources in a series of categories and requires the searcher to make a series of menu choices. For example, to find material on health care expenditure requires navigation from 'health and care', through to 'costs of healthcare and social service' and then to 'expenditure on healthcare'.

Beyond DoH and Office of National Statistics (ONS) statistics, there are sites that are useful for specific types of statistics. For communicable diseases the

Public Health Laboratory Service at <http://www.phls.co.uk/> offers detailed disease facts on specific diseases with an alphabetical index, and laboratory reports by geographical area since the early 1980s. The Communicable Disease Report Weekly is available in full text <http://www.phls.co.uk/publications/cdr.htm> and is an invaluable source for everyone concerned with the surveillance, prevention, and the control of human infection. Selected morbidity data (from a sample of general practices) is provided by the Royal College of General Practitioners <http://www.rcgp-bru.demon.co.uk/index.htm>. Relevant professional organisations, charities and special interest groups are also worth checking for specific statistical questions.

For researchers seeking access to the raw data of UK national surveys and censuses, the MIMAS site <http://www.mimas.ac.uk/datasets.html> is the key gateway. Similarly, the Data Archive at the University of Essex <http://www.data-archive.ac.uk/> allows users to identify whether any UK national health and health-related surveys have been undertaken on a particular subject. The site also provides links to other national data archives.

## Healthcare organisation and finance

The UK DoH Web sites, listed above, give some access to expenditure data. For example, figures on personal social services expenditure in England <http://www.doh.gov.uk/public/stats3.htm#expenditure> are available and English prescribing costs are given at <http://www.doh.gov.uk/stats/pca99.htm>. CMA Medical Data at <http://www.cmadata.co.uk/> provides UK tables with the numbers of hospital units and services and their capacity, whilst data on the quality and performance of NHS organisations are provided at <http://www.doh.gov.uk/nhsperformanceindicators/index.htm>. For statistical data relating to private healthcare in the UK, Laing and Buisson are the key source. Outline data, highlighting the number of people covered by private medical insurance is available at <http://www.privatehealth.co.uk/laing/pmi.htm>.

## Searching

Another approach to finding health statistics is to use general search engines (Lycos, AltaVista, etc.) or meta-search engines such as Dogpile <http://www.dogpile.com/> or Copernic 2000 <http://www.copernic.com/>.

A Copernic 2000 search on 'angina prevalence' across 8 UK-oriented search engines did produce some specific answers. Sifting through the results highlighted part of a guideline on angina with detailed incidence rates for angina by age and sex, and the Scottish Health Survey and Public Health Department Reports. However, a really useful source, the British Heart Foundation Health Promotion Research Group <http://www.dphpc.ox.ac.uk/bhfhprg/stats/index.html>

was not returned. Clearly, the source of data found by such searches needs to be verified by close reading of the documents and their references, but this approach did seem to provide a quick route into useful data, which had not been easily obtainable from national collections. Using several search phrases may also be required, such as 'angina incidence' or 'angina epidemiology'.

## Comparative health data

Comparing the performance and funding of the NHS with health services in other countries is highly topical and accessing sources of comparative data is possible through several sites. European statistics can be identified via the Resource Centre for Access to Data across Europe (r-Cade) <http://www-rcade.dur.ac.uk/> which provides links to collections and sites such as Eurostat. The OECD in Figures Web site <http://www.oecd.org/publications/figures/> offers comparative statistics on health expenditure, health status, and many non-health areas for countries in the OECD, as a taster for its non-Web publications. For comparative data on national disease control performance, life expectancy and public health the WHO World Health Report <http://www.who.int/whr/2000/en/report.htm> is a highly recommended source.

## Guides to sources and collections of statistics

There are literally hundreds of general guides and lists of statistics sites produced by organisations and academic libraries. One excellent list <http://www.lib.gla.ac.uk/ Depts/MOPS/Stats/medstats.html> (Fig. 4.3) has been compiled by Glasgow University Library. Equally, the SOSIG gateway provides a good set of statistics links <http://www.sosig.ac.uk/statistics/>. This is especially useful for locating non-UK information. If you are looking specifically for US health statistics, a good starting point is <http://www.links2go.com/topic/Health Statistics>. Statistical sources from a more financial perspective and with a US emphasis are listed on the HealthEconomics.com Web site <http://www.healtheconomics.com/ getSites.cfm?PAGE=Database>.

## Discussion groups

Discussion groups may also provide useful information and highlight current controversies. The Health Statistics User group is at <http://www.jiscmail.ac.uk/ lists/hsug.html> and the Radical Statistics Group list is at <http://www.jiscmail.ac.uk/ lists/radstats.html>.

## Summary

Regular searching for statistics will clearly generate your own personal list of useful sites. However, for very specific questions general search engines, restricting where possible to the country of interest, may be the quickest route

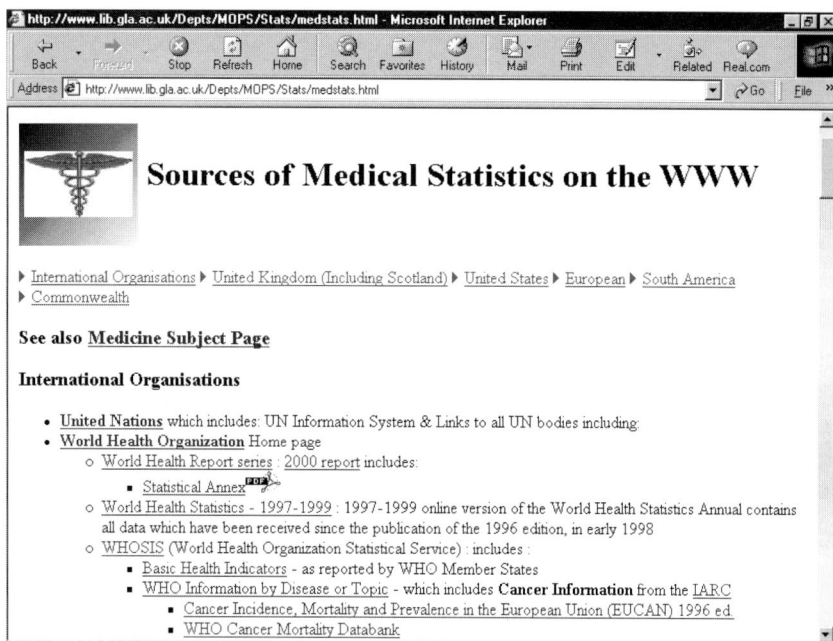

**Fig. 4.3** Glasgow University Library's list of medical statistics sites.

to useable data. If you retrieve information in this way the source and date of the data need to be investigated, so that they can be quoted with security. Moreover, finding the source of such data can help to direct you to the likely publisher of more recent data, much of which may still remain in paper form!

## References

1  Kiley R. Health statistics on the World Wide Web. *J R Soc Med* 1998; **91**: 264–5
2  Newman ML. *Health Statistics Sources: Searching Bibliographic Databases for Health Statistics*, 3rd edn. 1996. <http://www.nlm.nih.gov/nichsr/stats/database.html>
3  Kerrisen S, Macfarlane A (eds) *Official health statistics: an official guide*. London:Arnold, 2000

# 5

# Women's health on the Internet
## Part 1 – Pregnancy, childbirth and ultrasound

Hans van der Slikke

*Consultant Obstetrician/Gynaecologist at the*
*Free University Amsterdam Hospital*

hans@obgyn.net

## Health professionals

*Professional societies*

A good starting point for professionals is the site of the International Federation of Obstetrics & Gynaecology (FIGO) <http://www.figo.org>. FIGO is the umbrella for 101 national societies, of which more than 25 have their own Web sites, including the NVOG, the Obstetrics and Gynaecology Society for the Netherlands, <http://www.nvog.nl/> and the American College of Obstetrics and Gynecology <http://www.acog.org/>. These sites have a closed, members-only section as well as sections aimed at the general public. In the members area users can find clinical guidelines and topics devoted to specific areas of specialisation. In common with most professional organisations these pages also include a calendar of meetings, with regional information about accreditation of conferences and congresses.

The Web site of the UK Royal College of Obstetricians & Gynaecologists <http://www.rcog.org.uk/> contains guidelines, rules for medical audit and good clinical practice (Fig. 5.1). In contrast to other society sites, however, this information is visible for everybody: no hiding behind passwords! Crucially, individual recommendations have been graded according to the level of evidence on which they are based using a scheme endorsed by the NHS Executive. Such an approach is highly stimulating for professionals from all over the world who can compare these recommendations with their own guidelines.

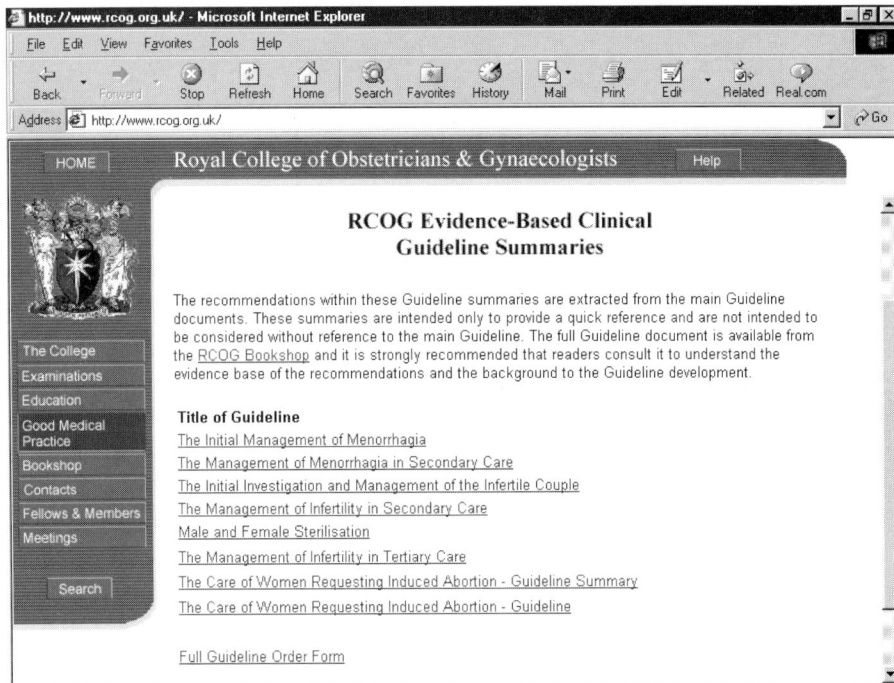

**Fig. 5.1** Evidence-based clinical summaries from the RCOG

## Other Web sites for O&G professionals

The premier gateway to information relating to obstetrics and gynaecology is OBGYN.net <http://www.obgyn.net/> (Fig. 5.2). Referred to as a 'Vortal' (vertical portal) OBGYN.net is the world's largest O&G Web site. The development of this gateway originates from the OB-GYN-L discussion list. The archives of this list are still available, and searchable from 1995, in the Medical Professional Forum <http://forums.obgyn.net/forums/ob-gyn-l/>.

At the OBGYN.net site clinical information has been divided into a number of featured sections. In the field of obstetrics these are Pregnancy and Childbirth, Fetal Monitoring, and Ultrasound. Each section has its own Editorial/Advisory Board. Recognising the international nature of the Internet, information in the professional section of the OBGYN.net site is published in five languages: English, Dutch, German, Portuguese and Spanish.

Although OBGYN.net is a sponsored Web site with several advertising banners, the editorial content is independent from their sponsors. OBGYN.net's original articles are peer reviewed by the Editorial Advisors of each section, and the site fully complies with principles devised by the Health on the Net Foundation <http:www.hon.ch/honcode/>.

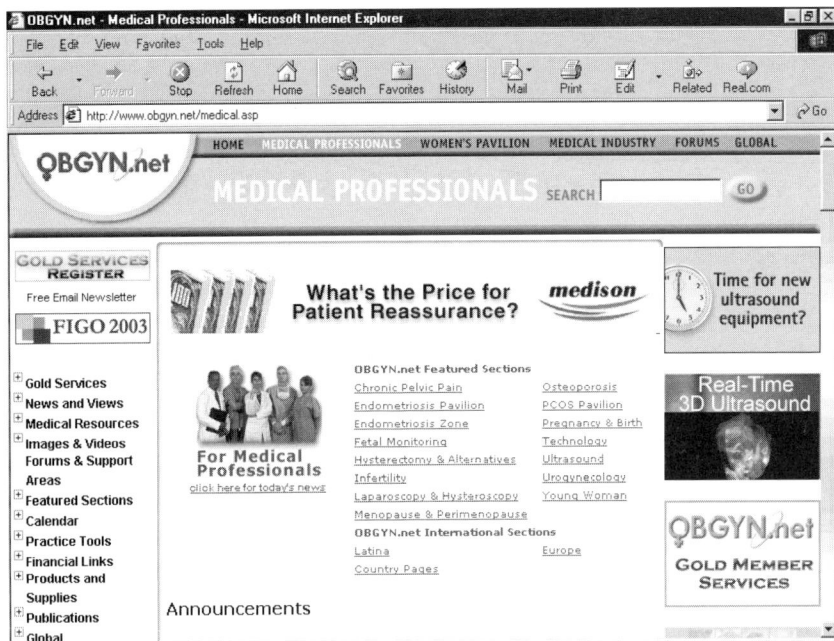

**Fig. 5.2** OBGYN.NET – the premier gateway to information on obstetrics and gynaecology

## Ultrasound

Within the ultrasound section of OBGYN.net <http://www.obgyn.net/us/us.asp/> obstetricians as well as sonographers can find case studies and an image gallery. Perhaps more originally users can also upload images to the gallery for purposes of consultation and analysis by experts from around the world. The ultrasound section has also started a peer-review system. Under this system only original papers, which have the approval of at least two reviewers, will be published. There is also a very active ultrasound forum for professionals <http://forums.obgyn.net/ultrasound/>. This generates around 100 postings a month and is another excellent way of seeking opinion from colleagues and peers.

From the ultrasound pages there are links to other obstetric ultrasound Web sites. However, rather than simply providing a hypertext link, all the suggested resources are described, rated (using a simple star system) and arranged in a clear hierarchical format to facilitate navigation. For example, within the section 'Ultrasound Clinical Information Links' resources are divided into categories such as *General Resources, Guidelines and Protocols,* and *Journals.*

The Fetus.net site <http://www.thefetus.net/> developed by Philippe Jeanty is dedicated to obstetric ultrasound. It contains more than 200 articles and around 900 images. One of the best parts is the 'Case of the Week' which takes the form of a clinical puzzle. Exciting and instructive in one! Recognising that some of the material on the site may be disturbing to a non-clinical audience, entrance to this site is only granted once you have accepted a disclaimer page and completed a simple registration form.

The American Institute of Ultrasound site <http://www.aium.org/> also has a lot of educational material and guidelines in ultrasound. This site is not only of use to obstetricians but also to other specialities who use ultrasound. Regrettably, the most interesting parts of this site are restricted to AIUM members.

The Web site of the International Society for Ultrasound in O&G (ISUOG) is also worth a visit <http://obg.med.wayne.edu/ISUOG/home.htm/> ISUOG has become the organisation for obstetricians, sonographers, and for fetal medicine specialists. The Web site contains information about forthcoming congresses and events, membership details and, of course, links. One of the links leads to the 'white' journal, namely the journal *Ultrasound in Obstetrics & Gynecology*. The contents of each issue are listed, but the full text is not available, even for members or subscribers.

Finally, the Fetal Echocardiography Web site <http://www.fetalecho.com/> developed by Greggory R. De Vore, provides information about the fetal echocardiography CD-ROM, and an online ordering form.

### Fetal monitoring

Information on the Web about fetal monitoring is relatively scarce. One useful starting point is the fetal monitoring section on the OBGYN.net site <http://www.obgyn.net/fm/fm.asp>. This sponsored section has several papers authored by some of world leading experts on cardiotocography (CTG) and fetal monitoring during labour. This site also includes information on other fetal monitoring devices, such as fetal pulse-oximetry.

At the site of the West Midlands Perinatal Institute, <http://www.wmpi.net/main.htm> developed for health professionals by Jason Gardosi, fetal growth and surveillance are the main topics. Gardosi, a founding member of ISIS (International Society of Intrapartum Surveillance) is also well known for his CTG-Tutor CD-ROM. For nurses new on the labour-ward and for young residents, the interpretation of CTGs gives a great deal of trouble. With the help of this educational tool, however, one can acquire a good basic knowledge and understanding of this subject. A demonstration version of the CTG-Tutor can be downloaded from this site at <http://www.wmpi.net/ctg/index_ctg.htm>.

### Midwifery resources

The American College of Nurse-Midwives <http://www.acnm.org> is the organisation of professional midwives in the United States. This site contains a wealth of professional information and educational material. Additional midwife practitioner resources can be found at <http://www.obgyn.net/pb/links/mp_midwife.htm>.

The real-life argument between doctors and midwives about the best way to deliver care continues in cyberspace. The Virtual Birth Centre <http://www.virtualbirth.com> and Carey Ann Ryan's Gentle Birth Midwife <http://www.gentlebirth.com> are examples of how one-sided the argument can become. Both of these sites, for example, are heavily in favour of home-births.

## Evidence-based obstetrics

Although obstetrics has a very long history as an empirical science, evidence-based obstetrics helps identify useless (and sometimes even harmful) procedures. A considerable part of the Cochrane Library comprises randomised trials in obstetrics. Indeed, the predecessor of the current Cochrane Library was the Cochrane Childbirth and Pregnancy Database. A selection of relevant abstracts in the current Cochrane Library can be found at <http://www.update-software.com/ccweb/cochrane/revabstr/g010index.htm>, but for obstetricians and gynaecologists the full text is available free of charge at <http//www.obgyn.net/cochrane.asp>.

## Consumers

Most of the Web sites of the professional organisations (highlighted above) have sections suitable for health consumers. This information will be written in a style and format suitable for a lay audience, and more importantly, be written in the native language of the health consumer. (The patient pages at the Netherlands Society for Obstetrics & Gynaecology <http://www.nvog.nl> are published in Dutch.)

## Pregnancy and childbirth

Consumers looking for medical information concerning pregnancy and birth will find the OBGYN.net section Pregnancy and Birth <http://www.obgyn.net/pb/pb.asp> a good place to start. One of the most popular corners is the Online Forum <http://forums.obgyn.net/pregnancy-birth> where women (and men) can ask questions concerning pregnancy problems. Questions are answered by professionals, often very quickly. All postings are archived and these can be searched to identify previous postings and their answers. There are also dedicated chat-hours on topics of interest to both pregnant women and new parents. Often, health professionals participate in these live forums.

Of the many commercial sites for pregnant women, Babycenter <http://www.babycenter.com/rcindex.html> is one of the most extensive. This is a clean and happy looking Web site with information on all aspects of pregnancy and childbirth. Would-be parents can use the preconception pages to learn about nutrition, prenatal health and even use the online ovulation calculator to determine fertile days. In contrast, parents who are coping with toddler temper tantrums can go to the Toddle pages <http://www.babycenter.com/toddler/> and read a number of articles on 'toddler discipline'.

Competing for the attention of pregnant women is The Labor of Love Web site <http://www.thelaboroflove.com> where a lot of attention is given to interactivity and the social and emotional side of pregnancy, rather than the medical aspects. In contrast, Childbirth.Org <http://www.childbirth.org/> adopts a more political approach. The information is presented from a non-clinical view, promoting pregnancy and birth as a natural process. There are fact-sheets covering a range of topics such as Caesarean sections <http://www. childbirth.org/section/CSFAQ.html> and natural remedies during pregnancy <http://www.childbirth.org/articles/remedy.html>. More classical and well-organised patient education material, where you can 'hear' the voices of US-obstetricians, can be found on the ACOG site at <http://www.acog.org>.

Sometimes things do not go the way they were expected: a miscarriage occurs or the baby dies. It is a known fact that support groups can become huge virtual communities, who will give comfort and consolation. A good gateway to this world is the Dealing with grief and loss Web site <http://members.tripod.com/

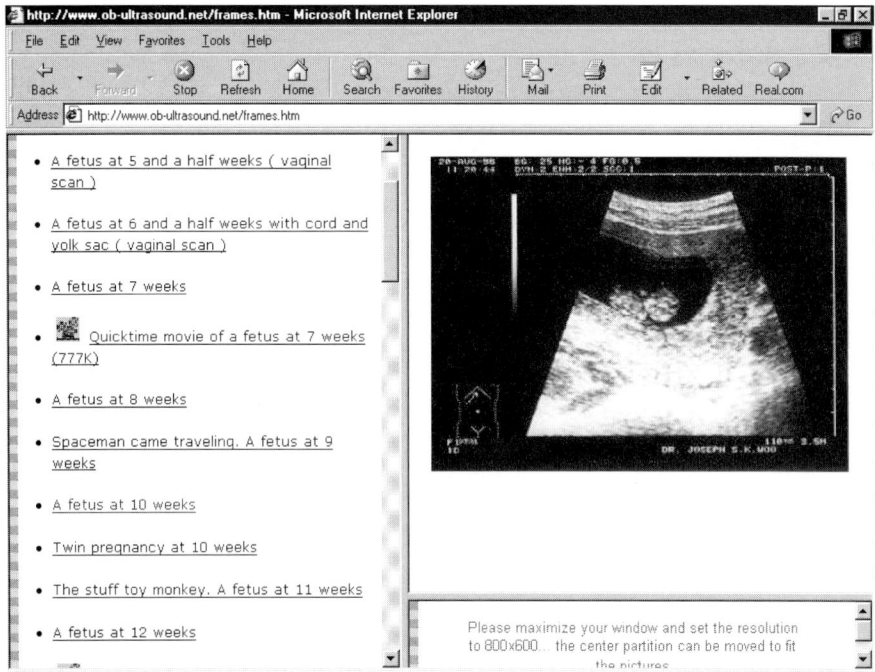

**Fig. 5.3** Joseph Woo's ultrasound site – a clear and comprehensive source of information

Crystalblue/loss.html>. From here there are links to sister organisations such as SIDS (Sudden Infant Death Syndrome) and MEND (Mommies Enduring Neonatal Death).

## Utrasound

Joseph Woo's ultrasound Web site <http://www.ob-ultrasound.net> has become a real classic (Fig. 5.3). This is a truly comprehensive site, with detailed information written in a way suitable for a lay audience. It gives clear explanation of all kinds of ultrasound procedures and a detailed history of obstetrical ultrasound. There are several links to other Web sites, where embryos and fetuses in all stages may be viewed.

## Conclusion

There is no shortage of information on the Internet relating to pregnancy, childbirth and ultrasound. Indeed, a search of AltaVista for the term 'pregnancy' returns more than one million Web pages. Recognising this problem, this article has attempted to provide a starting point to some of the best sites on the Web concerned with obstetrics and ultrasound. Part 2 of this article will adopt a similar approach but will focus on gynaecology and reproductive medicine.

# 6

# Women's health on the Internet
## Part 2: Gynaecology and reproductive

Hans van der Slikke

*Consultant Obstetrician/Gynaecologist at the*
*Free University Amsterdam Hospital*

hans@obgyn.net

## Introduction

The problems relating to searching the Internet for medical information are well known; too many sites are identified and there is no easy way to filter out the good from the bad. These problems are particularly pertinent when searching for information on topics such as fertility and contraception. For example, an AltaVista search for 'infertility' identifies a number of on-line 'donor catalogues' where users can select to buy eggs or sperm over the Internet based on details of the donor's height, weight, colour of eyes and medical history. Infamously, the Ron's Angels site introduced an auction for the ova and sperm of the most 'beautiful' donors in their catalogue. Not only are there considerable ethical issues here – should infertile couples pay for ova and sperm and, if so, should the price be dictated by the physical attractiveness of the donor? – but also practical considerations such as ensuring that the samples are not infected with HIV or hepatitis.

Consequently, if search engines are not the best place to start your exploration of the Web for information relating to gynaecology and reproductive medicine, where is? In my opinion, the best place to start is at the OBGYN.net site <http://www.obgyn.net> Since its launch in September 1996, OBGYN.net has become the gateway to information in the field of obstetrics and gynaecology. Moreover, it is one of the few Web sites that translates the content into other languages, like Spanish and Portuguese <http://latina.obgyn.net> and German and Dutch <http://europe.obgyn.net>.

Within the OBGYN.net site, there are several sections, each devoted to a gynaecological subspecialty. This is the approach I will adopt in the rest of this chapter.

## Fertility and infertility

FertiNet <http://www.ferti.net> is probably one of the best sites on the Web for infertility information (Fig. 6.1). The site has general information – including details of patient associations, fertility centres and treatment options – as well as more scientific information where practitioners in this field can identify the latest research, and learn about forthcoming conferences. Product information and access to on-line discussion forums is restricted to professional health workers in the field of assisted fertilisation and human reproduction.

The character of the site is mainly European and has a clear link to ESHRE, the European Society of Human Reproduction and Embryology <http://www.eshre.com>. ESHRE is one of the societies under the umbrella of the International Federation of Fertility Societies, IFFS <http://www.mnet.fr/webprofessionnel/i/iffs/index.htm>. At the IFFS site, you will find the usual information about the organisation, details of forthcoming conferences, and an on-line newsletter. Less typically, you will also find full text access (in PDF format) to a number of publications published

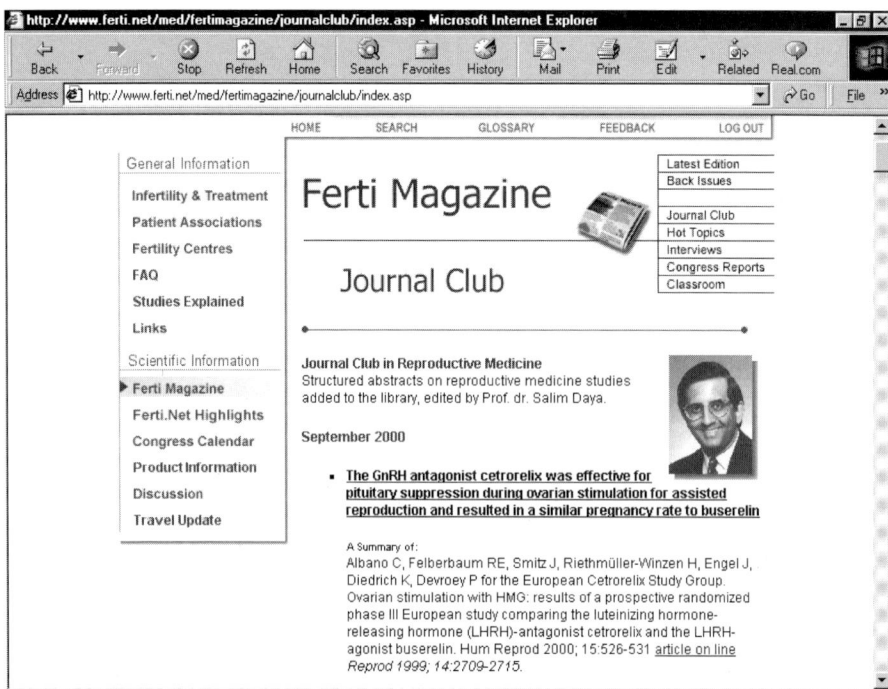

**Fig. 6.1** FertiNet – up-to-date information on all aspects of fertility

by this body including *Infertility and Contraception: A Textbook for Clinical Practice* <http://www.mnet.fr/webprofessionnel/i/iffs/bookinfertility/a_bookic.htm>.

Other useful resources include Dr Marc Perloe's IVF.com site <http://www.ivf.com> and the American Society for Reproductive Medicine <http://www.asrm.com>. Both sites include detailed FAQs for consumers, whilst the IVF.com site also has an on-line chat room, where Dr Perloe can be contacted at certain times of the week.

Self-help groups are another rich source of information. Resolve, the National Fertility Association, has an extensive Web site <http://www.resolve.org> that not only provides information about the key issues (such as how to select an infertility specialist), but through its on-line bulletin board and help lines it encourages visitors to communicate with other people who have similar concerns and worries. In the UK, the National Fertility Association <http://www.issue.co.uk/> provides a similar service.

## Contraception

For health professionals, the Web site of the International Planned Parenthood Federation <http://www.ippf.org> is a rich source of information. Of particular interest are the detailed country profiles <http://www.ippf.org/regions/countries/index.htm> which provide statistical data on fertility and contraception for over 180 countries. These profiles have been produced as a collaborative effort between Family Planning Associations affiliated to IPPF and IPPF Central and Regional Offices.

In the past few years, there has been much comment and debate about the link between combination oral contraceptives and cardiovascular disease. For an authoritative discussion on this topic, with clear conclusions and recommendations, the 1998 consensus document authored by the International Federation of Fertility Societies, should be consulted. The full-text of this is available at <http://www.mnet.fr/webprofessionnel/i/iffs/a_coc.htm>.

If contraception fails, abortion may be an option. This is obviously a very emotive subject, a fact reflected in many of the Web sites that address this issue. One Web site, however, that provides factual information without too much political colouring is the International Society of Abortion Doctors (ISAD) <http://alpha.nedernet.nl/~ngva/isadindex.htm>. Here, professionals will find a practical guide for doctors who undertake abortions and direct access to the ISAD-sponsored newsgroup <news//:sci.med.abortion>.

For consumers, the sites of the pharmaceutical companies like Organon <http://www.organon.com/>, Schering <http://www.femalelife.com/> and Ortho-McNeil <http://www.ortho-mcneil.com/> provide information about contraception. At the Ortho-McNeil site, for example, detailed information is provided on all the oral contraceptives, diaphragms and IUDs produced by this company. Information provided here ranges from quick fact sheets through to the full, and official, US Prescribing Information.

## Menopause

The North American Menopause Society (NAMS), a non-profit organisation 'devoted to promoting understanding of menopause, and thereby improving the health of women through midlife and beyond' has a wealth of information on its Web site <http://www.menopause.org/projour/abstract/mabstracts.html> For health professionals, on-line access is provided to abstracts from the journal *Menopause*, as well as online CME courses and details of scientific meetings. Consumers are not forgotten here either, as booklets, frequently asked questions, access to on-line discussion groups and details of clinicians who are members of NAMS, are all readily available.

Other sites of interest include the Doctor's Guide to Menopause <http://www. pslgroup.com/Menopause.htm> (Fig. 6.2) and the menopause and perimenopause sections on OBGYN.net <http://www.obgyn.net/meno/meno.asp>. Of particular interest here is the active forum, where specialists in this field answer patient's questions. Finally, readers should also be aware of the text *Practical HRT*, published by the European HRT network <http://www.hrtnet.org/prachrt/toc.htm>.

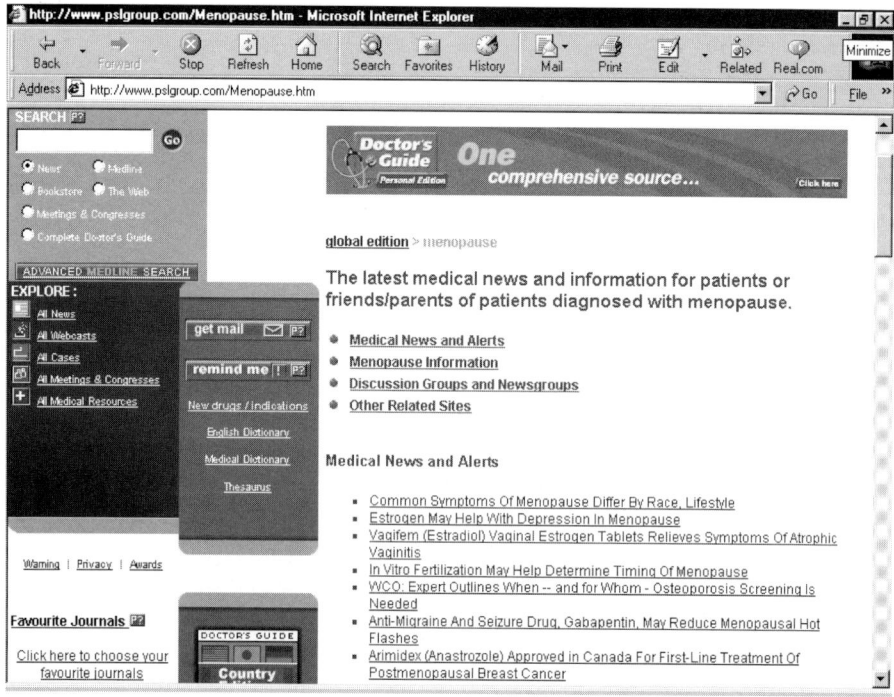

**Fig. 6.2** The Doctor's Guide to Menopause

This comprehensive and up-to-date textbook covers all the topics related to oestrogen replacement therapy.

## Laparoscopy and hysteroscopy

Starting again at OBGYN.net <http://www.obgyn.net/hysteroscopy/ hysteroscopy.asp> (Fig. 6.3) you will find on-line articles, case studies, fact sheets along with a collection of audio and video presentations that cover many aspects of laparoscopy and hysteroscopy.

The International Society for Gynecologic Endoscopy (ISGE) has an on-line gynaecologic endoscopic atlas <http://isge.org/pic/content.html>. Further images are available on the ENDOSURG site <http://www.chirurgie-endo.asso.fr/endosurg/ index.html>.

For information specifically on hysteroscopy, the Brasil Hysteroscopy site <http://www.histeroscopia.med.br/hysteroscopy.htm> developed by Dr Afonso, is worth visiting. Though it may not be the easiest site to navigate, there is much information to be found here including numerous on-line images and videos, and details of the history of hysteroscopy.

For clinical guidelines on the Web site for the Society for Obstetricians and Gynaecologists in Canada <http://www.sogc.org/SOGCnet/sogc_docs/common/

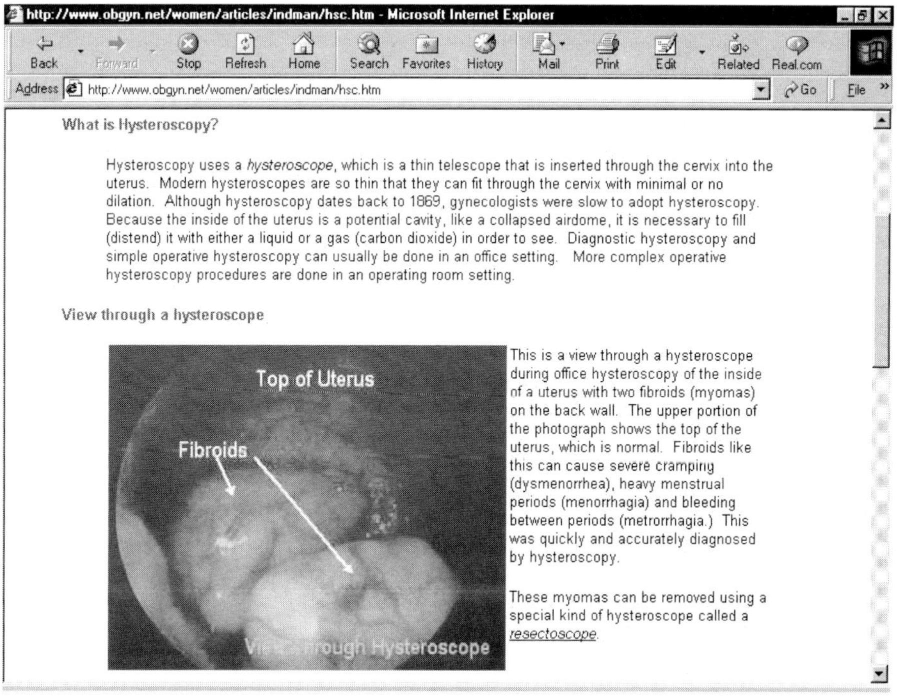

**Fig. 6.3** OBGYN.net authorative information for patients

guide/library e.shtml> is excellent reference point. If a guideline you seek is not covered here, the database of the National Guideline Clearing House <http://www.guidelines.gov/index.asp> can be searched.

## Urogynaecology

Patients who suffer from incontinence are, in general, embarrassed by their condition. For them, good information on the Web is essential. One site that addresses this need is Drylife <http://www.drylife.org/drylife.html>. Here, one is provided with a step-by-step guide to treating incontinence and access to a database of practising urologists.

For clinicians, the Web site of the American Urological Association <http://www.auanet.org/index hi.cfm> contains much useful information, including clinical guidelines, best-practice policies and access to the *Journal of Urology*. Much of this information, however, is only available to subscribing members.

The OBGYN.net section that deals with urogynaecology <http://www. obgyn.net/urogyn/urogyn.asp> contains original papers, congress videos and links, and is freely available.

## Oncology

Finally, I would like to highlight some sites that look at gynaecological oncology. (Note: although in some countries breast cancer falls within the remit of the gynaecological oncologist, it will not be discussed here.)

For oncology of the female genital organs, the FIGO (International Federation of Gynaecology and Obstetrics) staging is widely accepted. Information on the staging of the cancers of the uterus (cervix and corpus), ovary, vagina and vulva and gestational trophoblastic diseases (GTD) can all be downloaded from the FIGO site at <http://www.figo.org/default.asp?id=32>.

The US National Cancer Institute (NCI) has a wonderful site <http://www. nci.nih.gov> that contains general information about cancer and highly detailed location-specific information. (Information on location-specific cancer is accessible through the alphabetic listing of cancer-types <http://cancernet.nci.nih.gov/ alphalist.html>.)

Visitors to this site can also identify what clinical trials are currently being undertaken <http://cancernet.nci.nih.gov/trialsrch.shtml> on a particular cancer type. If a search yields too many trials, users are given the option of refining the search by stage of cancer, modality, and phase of trial. The NCI is also responsible for the CancerLit database, and to help clinicians make best use of this resource a number of pre-prepared searches have been constructed on all aspects of gynaecological cancers. Subjects covered include 'therapy of cervical cancer', 'gestational trophoblastic neoplasms' and 'vaginal and vulvar cancer'. Up-dated monthly, the searches and their results can be found at <http://cnetdb.nci.nih.gov/clinpdq/canlit/gynecologic.html>.

Other interesting sites relevant to this topic include the University of Washington Gynecologic Oncology Department <http://gynoncology.obgyn.washington.edu/> and Oncolink <http://www.oncolink.upenn.edu/> from the University of Pennsylvania. Both sites provide on-line tutorials on all the gynaecological cancer locations, whilst the University of Washington is particular strong on the treatment of rare gynaecological cancers.

For information about cervical pathology, the sites of the American Society for Colposcopy and Cervical Pathology <http://www.asccp.org/> and the National Cervical Cancer Coalition <http://www.nccc-online.org> are both highly recommended.

## Sites for patients and consumers

There is a strong belief that lay-people prefer information that is aimed at the health professional, perceiving it to be original and unfiltered information. This phenomenon is best illustrated by the enormous increase in the number of people searching MEDLINE since this database (PubMed) became freely available on the Web.

That said, there are still a number of very good Web sites that cover all aspects of women's health and focus exclusively on the lay consumer. The WellnessWeb Women's Health Centre <http://www.wellweb.com/WOMEN/women.htm> is one such example. WellnessWeb is a collaboration of patients, health care professionals, and other care-givers, whose mission is to 'help to find the best and most appropriate medical information and support available'.

Another useful site is Joan Korenman's home page <http://research.umbc.edu/~korenman/wmst/links_hlth.html> which provides a quick, annotated guide to some of the best sites that offer information about women's health issues.

Finally, MEDLINEplus <http://www.medlineplus.gov>, from the National Library of Medicine, provides additional authoritative information on a range of health issues, including women's health <http://www.nlm.nih.gov/medlineplus/womenshealth.html>. Recognising the difficulty, some users may experience in conducting an effective MEDLINE search, MEDLINEplus offers a number of pre-prepared 'clickable' MEDLINE searches.

## Conclusions

As this paper has shown, the Internet is positively awash with information about women's health. Indeed, a simple Google search for the phrase 'women's health' suggests that there are in excess of 896,000 pages on the Web that deal with this topic!

In an attempt to address this – and render such searches obsolete — this paper has attempted to direct the reader to the most interesting, relevant, and authoritative sites on the Web. Enjoy the ride!

# 7

# Human genome information on the Internet

Frank Norman

*Librarian at the National Institute for Medical Research*

fnorman@nimr.mrc.ac.uk

## Introduction

We are entering the age of molecular medicine[1]. In 1953 Watson and Crick famously described the structure of DNA[2] and laid the foundations for the new science of Molecular Biology, thereby profoundly affecting the direction of medical research. In particular, the establishment of the Human Genome Project (HGP) in the late 1980s led to an astonishing increase in the amount of information available about human genetics[3]. The first rough draft of the genome has recently been completed and on current plans the Project will complete an accurate, high-quality sequence of the human genome by 2003[4], the 50th anniversary of that famous paper. However, the debate on how this new scientific knowledge will or should affect medical practice has only just begun[5]. Patients and general practitioners alike are at the beginning of a steep learning curve. It has recently been stated that 'a broad educational effort is needed to increase awareness of the scope and potential of genetic information among health professionals and the public'[6].

The Internet is a rich source of genetic information. Biological researchers were early users of the Internet and over the past decade a huge array of research information has been made available on the Internet. The founders of the Human Genome Project also recognised that the successful completion of their program would raise many contentious non-scientific issues and one part of the project is devoted to ethical, legal and social issues (ELSI). More recently the burgeoning consumer health informatics movement[7,8] has brought a variety of patient-oriented genetic information resources.

47

This chapter will look at the genomics information on the Web, focusing on resources that are available to researchers, healthcare professionals and to patients and the general public.

## Sites for researchers

The most well-known site for molecular biology and genomic information is Entrez <http://www.ncbi.nlm.nih.gov/Entrez/>, from the US National Center for Biotechnology Information (NCBI). Entrez provides access to the major gene and protein sequence databanks, such as GenBank and Swiss-Prot, integrated with gene maps, protein structure information data sets of population sequences, and with literature references in MEDLINE. Related records are extensively cross-linked, to allow researchers to follow logical links between maps and gene sequences, gene sequences and protein sequences, or protein sequences and protein structures. Graphical views of genetic maps and 3-dimensional protein structures are also available. There are several other useful resources on the NCBI Web-site, all linked from the home page. RefSeq and LocusLink are part of the Reference Sequence project which will provide reference sequence standards for the naturally occurring molecules – from chromosomes to mRNAs to proteins. Coffee Break is a collection of brief reports of recent biological discoveries, using interactive tutorials to demonstrate the role that bioinformatics tools played in the research process. The Education section of the site includes tutorials on using Entrez, sequence similarity searches and other NCBI tools as well as the text of a very well-produced course on Molecular Biology Information run by the Medical Library Association.

The Expasy molecular biology server <http://www.expasy.ch/> is the leading site for protein information. It is the home of Swiss-Prot, a curated protein sequence database which provides a high level of annotation about each protein, a minimal level of redundancy and a high level of integration with other databases. The site also provides several other protein databanks, tools for protein modelling and the burgeoning field of proteomics research, as well as 3-dimensional images of proteins and other biological macromolecules.

The European Bioinformatics Institute (EBI) <http://www.ebi.ac.uk>, based at Hinxton Hall near Cambridge, is an outstation of the European Molecular Biology Laboratories. Its central activity is the production of the EMBL Nucleotide Sequence Database, and it provides a Web interface to this databank using the Sequence Retrieval System (SRS). The site also gives access to more than 70 other more specialised databanks using the same interface, allowing multiple resources to be searched with a single query (Fig. 7.1). A collection of tools for and information about microarray informatics, which is set to become an important field for biology, are also included. The EBI in collaboration with the

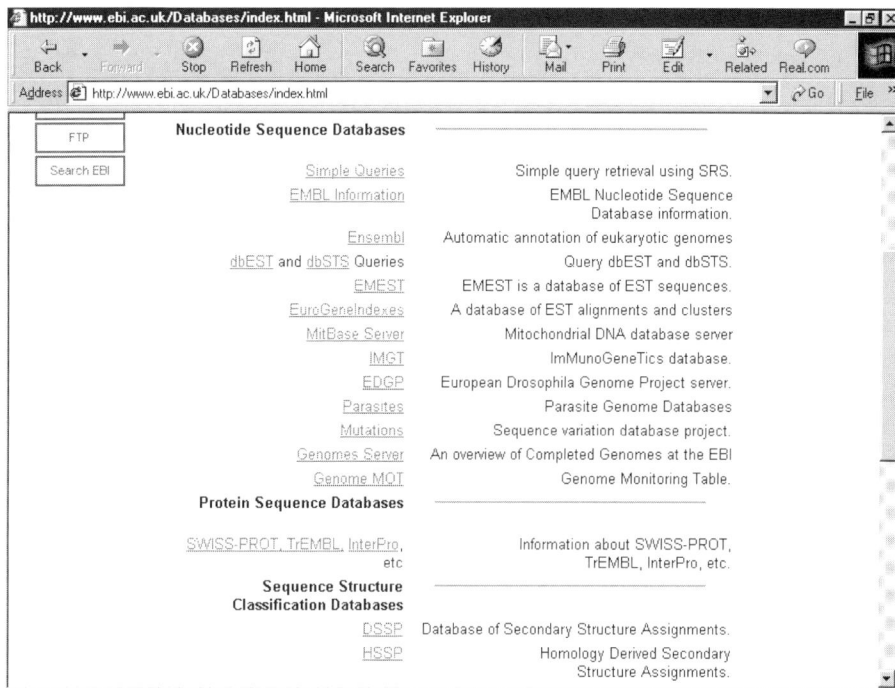

**Fig. 7.1** Range of bioinformatic databases from the EBI

Sanger Centre are developing the Ensembl project <http://www.ensembl.org/>, a software system designed to automate the management and annotation of genome information (Fig. 7.2). It also provides a reference view of genome sequence data.

The MRC's Human Genome Mapping Project Resource Centre (HGMP-RC), also based at Hinxton, is the focus of the UK gene mapping community. Its Web site <http://www.hgmp.mrc.ac.uk> offers access to many sequence resources through a variety of interfaces (some available only to registered users). It also contains the GenomeWeb, a subject gateway to other Web sites for genome researchers, and lecture notes from HGMP-RC courses in the use of computing and molecular biology.

A collection of articles about molecular biology databases is published every January in *Nucleic Acids Research* along with a list of resources[9]. This list is available on the journal's Web site, <http://intl-nar.oupjournals.org/cgi/content/full/28/1/1> with links into each database mentioned. It is an excellent way to catch up on database activity and trends in this field, though the sheer quantity of resources and their increasing specialisation is pretty daunting these days.

There are several good books aimed at those struggling to use bioinformatics tools for the first time. The authors of one of the best[10] have produced a Web site called 'Protein sequence analysis: a practical guide' <http://www.biochem.ucl.ac.uk/bsm/dbbrowser/jj/prefaxefrm.html>.

## Sites for healthcare professionals

The ever-reliable Virtual Hospital, based in Iowa, USA, provides a series of substantial multimedia textbooks, and in 1998 they added *Clinical Genetics: A Self Study for Health Care Providers* <http://www.vh.org/Providers/Textbooks/ClinicalGenetics/Contents.html>. It consists of four lessons 'designed to increase your knowledge about genetics and teach you skills to identify and refer families for evaluation'.

The UK Department of Health maintains a site devoted to genetics in healthcare <http://www.doh.gov.uk/genetics.htm>. It provides information about the major relevant UK government advisory groups, and a link to the Human Genetics Commission (HGC) Web site. The HGC is the UK Government's advisory body on how 'new developments in human genetics will impact on people and healthcare, with a particular focus on social and ethical issues'. Its Web site <http://www.hgc.gov.uk/> contains information about the HGC, its work plan, minutes of meetings and an explanation of the regulatory framework. I also links to the Web sites of the bodies that proceeded it, notably the Human Genetics Advisory Commission where the full-text of reports on genetic testing and on cloning, can be found.

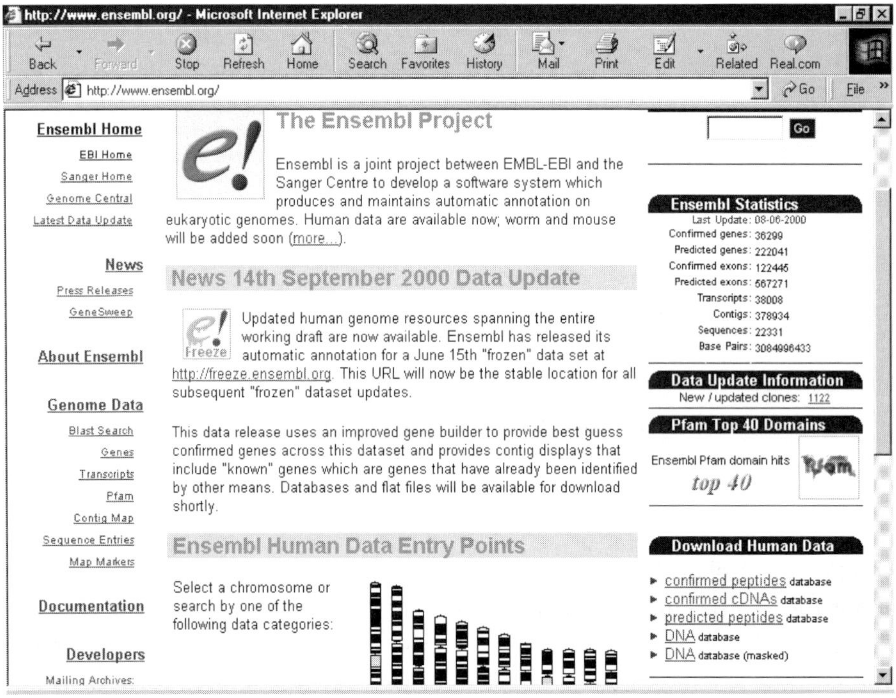

**Fig. 7.2** Ensembl – managing and annotating genome information

Guide to Healthcare Resources on the Internet

The Public Health Genetics Unit is an NHS-funded centre whose aim is to bring together policy makers, health service professionals, academic researchers and consumer stakeholders to think about what genetics will mean for the future of the health service. Its Web site <http://www.medinfo.cam.ac.uk/phgu> is an excellent and frequently updated resource containing news and information about advances in genetics, their impact on public health and the prevention of disease. It includes a newsletter that highlights interesting papers and reviews, a database of publications and organisations, and a comprehensive set of links to external sites containing information about genetics and genomics.

Online Mendelian Inheritance in Man (OMIM) <http://www3.ncbi.nlm.nih.gov/Omim/> is a comprehensive and authoritative resource which is linked with many other related genome and molecular biology information resources on the Web. OMIM is a catalogue of human genes and genetic disorders, with over 10,000 entries, authored and edited by Dr Victor A. McKusick and colleagues at Johns Hopkins University and elsewhere. It is intended for use 'primarily by physicians and other professionals concerned with genetic disorders, by genetics researchers and by advanced students in science and medicine'. The database is a compilation of review articles each concerned with a specific disease or syndrome, detailing the most recent genetic research. It is extensively referenced.

GeneClinics <http://www.geneclinics.org/> is 'a peer-reviewed clinical genetic information resource consisting of concise descriptions of specific inherited disorders and authorative, current information on the role of genetic testing in the diagnosis, management, and counselling of patients with these inherited conditions'.

The British Society for Human Genetics is a forum for professionals working in all aspects of Human Genetics, from cutting edge research to the delivery of genetics services'. Their Web site <http://www.bshg.org.uk/> includes information about the society and its activities, statements on topical issues, reports and documents. There is also a listing of Regional Genetics Centres in the UK.

## Sites for the general public and patients

The best source of information about the Human Genome Project is the Oak Ridge National Laboratory site, funded by the US Department of Energy <http://www.ornl.gov/hgmis/>. It contains a wide variety of basic information about the project and its progress, and selected links to resources elsewhere. Three valuable and well-illustrated publications on this site cater for varying levels of understanding, from expert to novice: *Primer on Molecular Genetics*, *To Know Ourselves* and *Your Genes, Your Choices*.

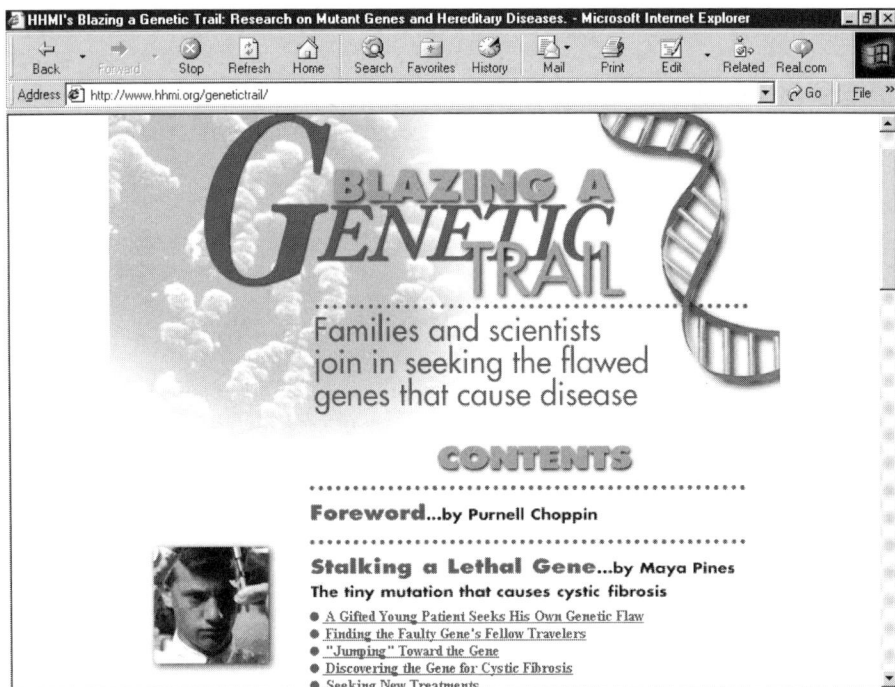

**Fig. 7.3** Howard Hughes Medical Institute – blazing a genetic trail

Closer to home, the Wellcome Trust Web site includes a section on the Genome Project <http://www.wellcome.ac.uk/en/genome/>, with commentaries on the completion of the first draft and a history of the UK Human Genome Project.

The (US) National Information Resource on Ethics & Human Genetics Web site <http://www.georgetown.edu/research/nrcbl/nirehg.htm> provides useful explanations of gene therapy, genetic testing, eugenics and the Human Genome Project, all well-referenced and updated.

The US Public Broadcasting System produced a TV program on 'A Question of Genes: Inherited Risks'. It featured seven stories exploring individual experiences with genetic testing and the resulting choices. The associated Web site <http://www.pbs.org/gene/> contains transcripts of the case studies and further background information.

Blazing a Genetic Trail, <http://www.hhmi.org/genetictrail/> (Fig. 7.3), published by the Howard Hughes Medical Institute in Maryland, USA is a survey of the current state of genetic medicine, well illustrated and clearly written in an engaging style.

The Genetic Interest Group (GIG) is a UK alliance of organisations which support those affected by genetic disorders. GIG aims to promote the awareness and understanding of genetic diseases by providing information on genetics services in the UK. Their Web site <http://www.gig.org.uk/> contains the full text of many publications for patients and their families and several policy documents issued by GIG on topical issues or in response to consultation documents.

Contact-a-Family is a UK charity 'dedicated to helping families who care for children with any disability or special need'. Their Web site <http://www. cafamily.org.uk/index.html> includes much helpful background about genetics, a glossary, lists of organisations and the CaF Directory of Specific Conditions and Rare Syndromes. The CaF Directory provides a description of each condition and details of relevant support groups.

An index to support groups in the US is available from the University of Kansas, Genetic Conditions/Rare Conditions Support Groups & Information Page <http://www.kumc.edu/gec/support/>. This provides contact details for support groups, but also has many links to relevant patient information Web sites for each condition.

The NCBI's 'Genes and Disease' site <http://www.ncbi.nlm.nih.gov/disease/> contains profiles of disease genes and is aimed at students and the general public. Diseases are arranged in categories (e.g. cancer, immune system etc.) and there is an easily understandable explanation of each disease that is included, plus links into more specialist resources. There is also a chromosome browser, allowing you to view an image of a chromosome and see what diseases are associated with it.

## More and more

In this survey of human genome information on the Internet I have only been able to give a brief impression of what is available. The sites described cover a broad spectrum of interests and present a huge amount of data, but beyond them are many more specialised resources from growing fields such as protein structure, functional genomics and non-human genomes. It is a frighteningly large and complex assemblage of information, but even more frightening is the certainty that it will become larger and more complex as research progresses!

There was a time when you could talk about 'Information' without mentioning the Internet, but that seems incredible now. The Internet has transformed our ideas about information availability and our habits of information use. Medicine is today undergoing a similar transformation, as genetic concepts and explanations become incorporated in our understanding of physiology, disease and behaviour. New clinical problems and ethical worries are already presenting themselves as a result. Researchers, clinicians and patients face great challenges in accessing and understanding the results of the Human Genome Project. The Internet will be an invaluable aid in facing up to these challenges.

### References

1. Bell J. The human genome. In: *Clinical Futures*. Marinker M, Peckham M, eds. 1998, London:BMJ Publishing Group.
2. Watson JD, Crick FHC, A structure for deoxyribose nucleic acid. *Nature* 1953; **171**: 737–8.
3. Watson JD. The Human Genome Project: past, present and future. *Science* 1990; **248**: 44–9.
4. Pennisi E. Finally, the Book of Life and instructions for navigating it. *Science* 2000; **288**: 2304–7.
5. Gill M, Richards T. Meeting the challenge of genetic advance. *BMJ* 1998; **316**: 570.
6. Kinmonth AL et al. The new genetics. Implications for clinical services in Britain and the United States. *BMJ* 1998; **316**:767–70.
7. Eysenbach G. Consumer health informatics. *BMJ* 2000; **320**: 1713–6.
8. Ferguson T. Health online and the empowered medical consumer. *Joint Commission Journal on Quality Improvement* 1997; **23**: 251–7.
9. Baxevanis AD. The molecular biology database collection: an online complilation of relevant database resources. *Nucleis Acids Res* 2000; **320**: 1713–6.
10. Attwood TK, Parry-Smith DJ. *Introduction to bioinformatics*. London: Addison, Wesley Longman, 1999.

# 8

# Cancer information on the Internet

Simon Cotterill

*North of England Children's Cancer Research Unit*

Simon@SimonCotterill.com

## Introduction

Approximately 1 in 3 people will develop cancer during their lifetime. Along with heart disease, cancer is the leading cause of death in Western populations. It is not surprising, therefore, that the rapid growth in the use of the Internet has been associated with a vast and ever growing amount of online cancer related information. Cancer organisations, cancer centres, pharmaceutical companies, support groups and individuals all compete to provide information for health professionals, patients and their carers.

Ready access to health information has the potential to empower the patient. Indeed, research suggests that patients who play an active role in decisions about their treatments have improved health outcomes[1]. Cancer e-mail discussion lists also enable patients to communicate and share experiences with others in similar circumstances. However, since the early days of the Web concerns have been voiced about quackery and unverified health claims relating to alternative cancer treatments[2,3]. There are a number of proposed standards for health information on the Internet, but ultimately they are unenforceable; more education about quality of information issues is needed.

For health professionals and researchers the Internet provides access to a variety of medical databases and a gateway to the latest oncology research. It may be used to encourage the more rapid dissemination of new techniques and standards[4]. The Internet also offers incredible potential for connecting those with similar research interests from around the world.

Whether physicians have the time or inclination to use the Internet is another question. However, even those who do not use the Internet are likely to be affected by it. Increasingly, medical teams are counselling patients who download medical information from the Internet[5]. Such teams may also witness an increase in 'protocol shopping' by patients who use the Web to find out about different protocols and clinical trials[6].

In this article, I will highlight some of the most important cancer resources on the Internet, dividing these resources into four main areas: (i) sites for the specialist; (ii) resources relevant to medical education and teaching; (iii) cancer sites for patients and the public; and (iv) further information.

## Specialist cancer sites

The American National Cancer Institute (NCI) <http://www.nci.nih.gov/> has a range of services which offer some of the most comprehensive online oncology information. The best known of these is CancerNet <http://cancernet.nci.nih.gov/> which includes PDQ, NCI's comprehensive cancer database of peer-reviewed summaries on cancer treatment, screening, prevention, and supportive care. Statements are reviewed on a monthly basis by a panel of medical experts (Fig. 8.1). Cancernet is distributed to several sites around the world, including the

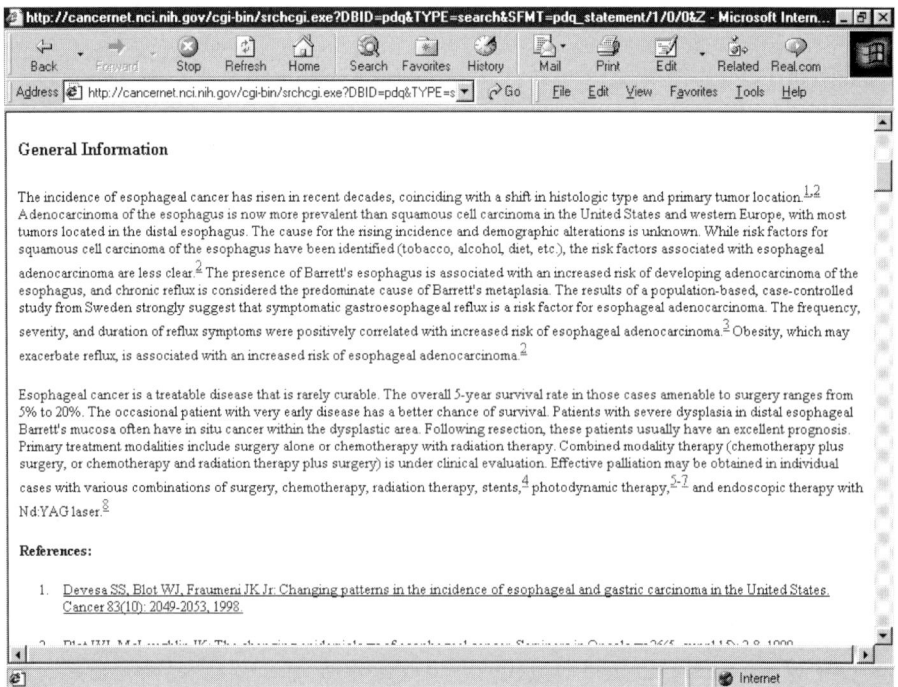

**Fig. 8.1** PDQ – latest information reviewed and updated by cancer experts

Gray Laboratory Cancer Research Trust in the UK <http://www.graylab.ac.uk/cancernet.html>.

CancerLit <http://cnetdb.nci.nih.gov/cancerlit.shtml> is a bibliographic database maintained by the NCI. It is ideal for specialist searches as it incorporates a wider range of material than MEDLINE, with conference abstracts, books, reports, and doctoral theses included as well as journal citations. It is up-dated with more than 8000 records every month.

OncoLink <http://oncolink.upenn.edu/> was one of the first large cancer Web sites. It is produced by the University of Pennsylvania Cancer Center and has extensive resources for both public and health professionals for a wide range of cancer types and medical specialities. The new OncoLinkTV section includes online videos about specific cancers; future-looking but a transatlantic download via a slow modem can be rather challenging.

The Cancer Genome Anatomy Project <http://www.ncbi.nlm.nih.gov/ncicgap/> is an NCI funded site which includes a directory of oncogenes and tumour suppressor genes. Records are linked with Entrez, UniGene, OMIM and other major gene databases. The site includes data and information about initiatives such as the Human Tumour Gene Index, Molecular Fingerprinting Initiative, Cancer Chromosome Aberration Project and the Genetic Annotation Initiative.

The International Union Against Cancer Web site <http://www.uicc.org/> provides information about UICC programs, publications and lists member organisations around the world. This site has one of the best facilities for identifying oncology conferences and meetings. They will also host, free of charge, Web pages about forthcoming oncology conferences.

Cancer Mondial <http://www-dep.iarc.fr/> is produced by the Unit of Descriptive Epidemiology at the International Agency for Research on Cancer and provides access to population based cancer statistics (Fig. 8.2). It hosts three large databases: EUCAN90, The WHO Cancer Mortality Databank and GlobalCan. The latter is a JAVA application which allows the user to generate tables and graphs for particular cancers/countries.

## Medical education and teaching resources

OncoLink (referenced above) is a particularly good site for online case studies. For example, the section on paediatric oncology has a case of the month which draws together radiological, histopathological and clinical data for discussion. It also features a radiation oncology teaching resource.

The Web site of the University of Texas M.D. Anderson Cancer Center <http://rpiwww.mdacc.tmc.edu/mmlearn/> has a significant multimedia and learning resources section. This includes the NetCME Oncology Imaging and

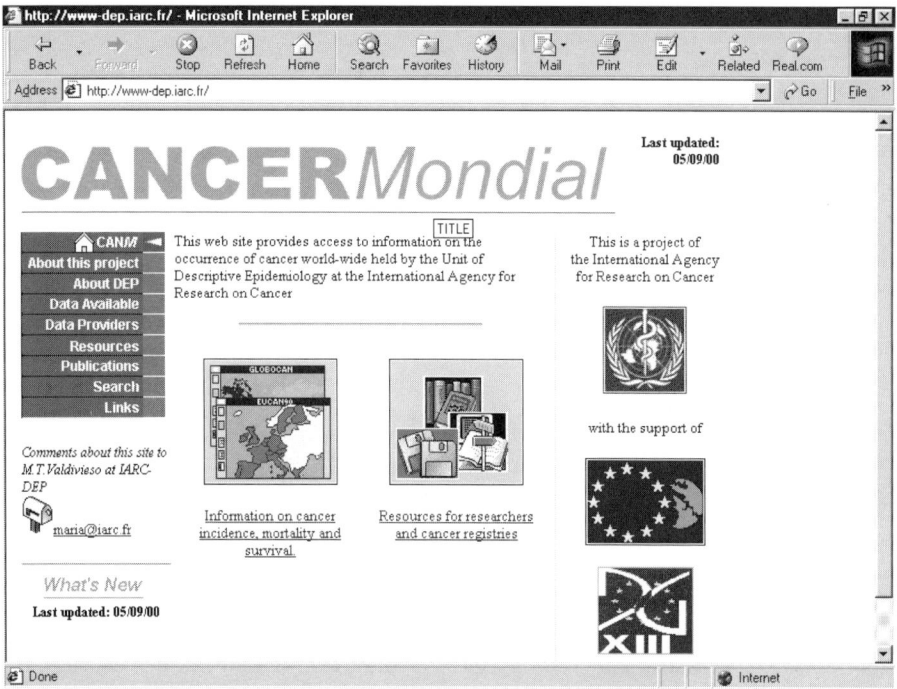

**Fig. 8.2** Cancer statistics from the IARC

Diagnosis site, which is a collaborative international network of image servers. The service is available in several languages and those with paid registration can gain CME Credits, awarded by the American Medical Association.

A number of sites also have slides suitable for oncology teaching which can be down-loaded free of charge. The BioOncology Online Resource Centre <http://www. biooncology.com/>, for example, includes a range of teaching aids which focus on the many aspects of biological oncology. There are also pathology and radiology sites which contain large numbers of oncology images and referenced case studies. Examples include WebPath <http://www.medstat.med.utah.edu/WebPath/ webpath.html>, the Urbana Atlas of Pathology <http://www.med.uiuc.edu/PathAtlasf/ titlepage.html> and the Radiology Museum <http://www.sbu.ac.uk/~dirt/museum/ museum.html>.

## Cancer sites for patients and the public

The British Association for Cancer United Patients (BACUP) Web site <http://www. cancerbacup.org.uk/> provides detailed information for many types of cancers. Though this information is authored by oncologists, it is presented in a format that is suitable for the lay person. Using the 'Patients Menu' there are a large number of online booklets for many types of cancer. There is also a searchable database of UK cancer support groups. Another British site, CancerHelp UK <http://www.cancerhelp.org.uk> also provides a patient-oriented information service. This site is produced by the Cancer Research Campaign Institute for Cancer Studies at the University of Birmingham.

For more cancer-specific information, the Imperial Cancer Research Fund (ICRF) <http://www.icnet.uk/> is a good starting point. This site also contains details of on-going research, oncology news and a useful child-oriented guide to cells entitled *Cells Are Us*. Another good source of information is the Leukaemia Research Fund site <http://www.lrf.org.uk/>. This has numerous online booklets and leaflets, many of which contain information about many of the rarer haematological malignancies.

The Association of Cancer Online Resources (ACOR) is a US patient-driven organisation. Their Web site <http://www.acor.org/> provides a mirror of CancerNet and hosts a number of patient produced sites for specific cancers (haematological, colon, testicular, pancreatic, breast and children's cancers). ACOR also hosts over 70 cancer e-mail lists many of which are self-styled online support groups.

The Harvard Center for Cancer Prevention has produced a site called Your Cancer Risk <http://www.yourcancerrisk.harvard.edu>. This interactive site allows users to assess their risk for a number of common types of cancer and offers personalised tips for lowering their chance of developing cancer.

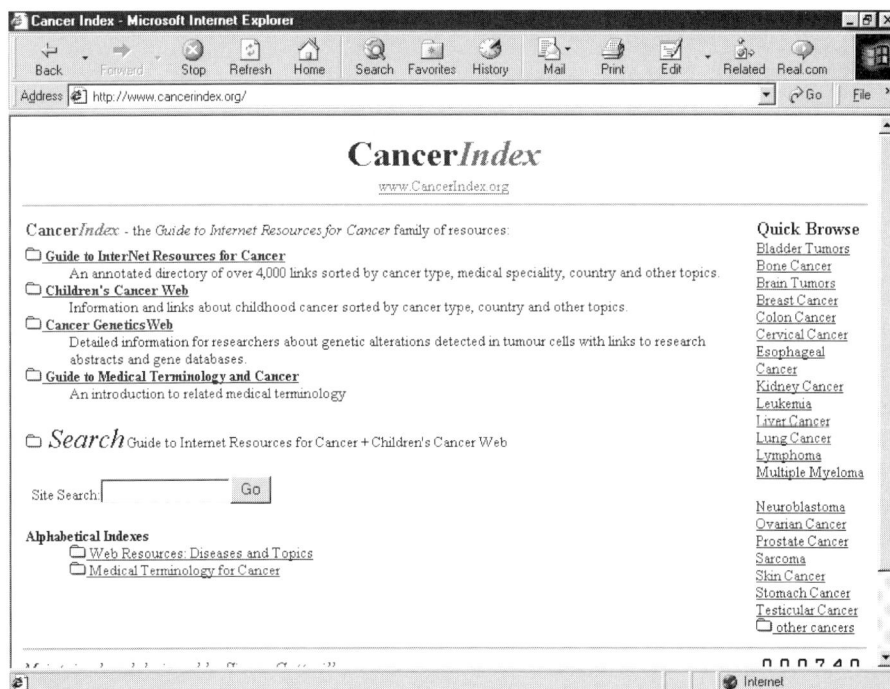

**Fig. 8.3** Cancer index – gateway to cancer resources on the Internet

# Further information

The resources listed here only scratch the surface of what is available. In particular, there are many disease and speciality-specific sites which publish expert information and run specialist forums. As a starting point for further exploration I have compiled a *Guide to Cancer Information on the Internet* <http://www.cancerindex.org/>. This single resource contains reviewed links to more than 4000 cancer Web sites. To facilitate navigation, the links are sorted by disease type, medical speciality, country and other topics (Fig. 8.3). Separate interfaces are provided for health professionals, researchers and patients.

The Internet has changed the availability and accessibility of cancer information forever. In the past, a patient's physician was usually their sole channel for information about cancer. Now patient guides and medical texts from around the world are only a click away. While this presents new challenges, it also provides great potential benefits to both professional and lay audiences.

## References

1   Greenfield S, Kaplan S. Ware Jr JE. Expanding patient involvement in care: effects on patient outcomes. *Ann Intern Med* 1985; **102**: 520–8
2   Keoun B. Cancer patients find quackery on the Web. *J Natl Cancer Inst* 1996; **88**: 1263–5
3   Bower H. Internet sees growth of unverified health claims. *BMJ* 1996; **313**: 381
4   Keoun B. At last, doctors begin to jump online. *J Natl Cancer Inst* 1996; **88**: 1610–2
5   Glode LM. Challenges and opportunities of the Internet for medical oncology. *J Clin Oncol* 1996; **14**: 2181–6
6   Vaitones V *et al*. Protocol 'shopping' on the Internet. *Cancer Practice* 1995; **3**: 274–8

# 9

# Nursing information on the Internet

Rod Ward

*Lecturer in the Department of Acute and Critical Care School of Nursing and Midwifery, University of Sheffield, Sheffield, UK*

rod.ward@sheffield.ac.uk

## Introduction

Despite greater numbers of practitioners, nursing resources on the Internet are not as extensive as those for physicians. This situation is possibly the consequence of pre-existing levels of IT knowledge and skills, and possibly because of gender, power and financial issues. Recent years, however, have seen the move of nursing education into higher education with a subsequent improvement in IT resources and network access. Equally encouraging is the recognition by NHS Trusts of the importance of the Internet as a medium for staff education and development.

Nursing information on the Internet has increased rapidly over the last few years. In 1993, when I first started using the Internet, I could find only four Web sites that had a nursing focus. Also, as there was no single index to nursing resources, I created my own Web site of Nursing and Health Care Resources on the Net <http://www.shef.ac.uk/~nhcon>. This site now points to over 2000 nursing resources and it is by no means comprehensive! In addition to the Web, there are also hundreds of mailing lists and several news groups devoted to nursing and nursing issues.

In this article, I give an overview of Internet resources that are of practical use to today's nurse.

## Web sites

Nursing Web sites range from those concerned with a particular aspect of clinical practice or nursing speciality, to regulatory bodies and online journals.

61

Though the Internet is a global medium, in an attempt to balance the US dominance I have chosen some UK examples.

Any nurse practising in the UK who needs to check out issues relating to registration or 'Post Registration Education and Practice Project' (PREPP) will find the United Kingdom Central Council for Nursing, Midwifery and Health Visiting <http://www.ukcc.org.uk/> a good place to start. This Web site has information about the council and how it works, along with a collection of circulars and publications. Equally useful is the English National Board Web site <http://www.enb.org.uk>, which contains information about the work of the Board along with a searchable database of relevant publications.

Keeping up-to-date with current developments and research is a responsibility all nurses must undertake. To assist in this task there are now several nursing journals that are available on the Internet. These either appear as electronic versions of paper journals or as online journals with no paper equivalent.

The *Nursing Standard On-Line* <http://www.nursing-standard.co.uk> was the first weekly nursing journal to have a Web presence. Though it does not contain the full text of all the articles in the paper version, it does include the contents pages, news items and advertisement sections. A feature of particular interest is the online news section – which carries material typically about nursing and the Internet and keyword Internet searches – that is not available in the paper version. This has now been joined by the other major weekly UK nursing journal, *Nursing Times* <http://www.nursingtimes.net/>.

A journal that is only available on the Web is *World Wide Wounds* <http://www.smtl.co.uk/World-Wide-Wounds/>. Published by the Surgical Materials Testing Laboratory, this journal provides information on wound management strategies and products. It now also has a Web based discussion forum for wound management related topics.

There are also numerous Web sites organized by practitioners working in particular clinical areas. For example, the *Nurse Practitioner* <http://www.healthcentre.org.uk/np/> Web site has information about how this role is developing in the UK. The site also hosts a discussion list where ideas can be discussed and common problems solved.

Nurses working in operating departments should also be aware of the Web site established by the UK National Association of Theatre Nurses <http://www.natn.org.uk/>. This site has a range of educational resources (*NATN Journal*, details of publications, etc.) and a fairly extensive jobs' forum. Less specifically, any nurse who has to deal with either acute or chronic pain should visit Dee's Pain Management <http://www.web-shack.com/dee/> Web site, which has information on topics such as patient-controlled analgesia (PCA) and

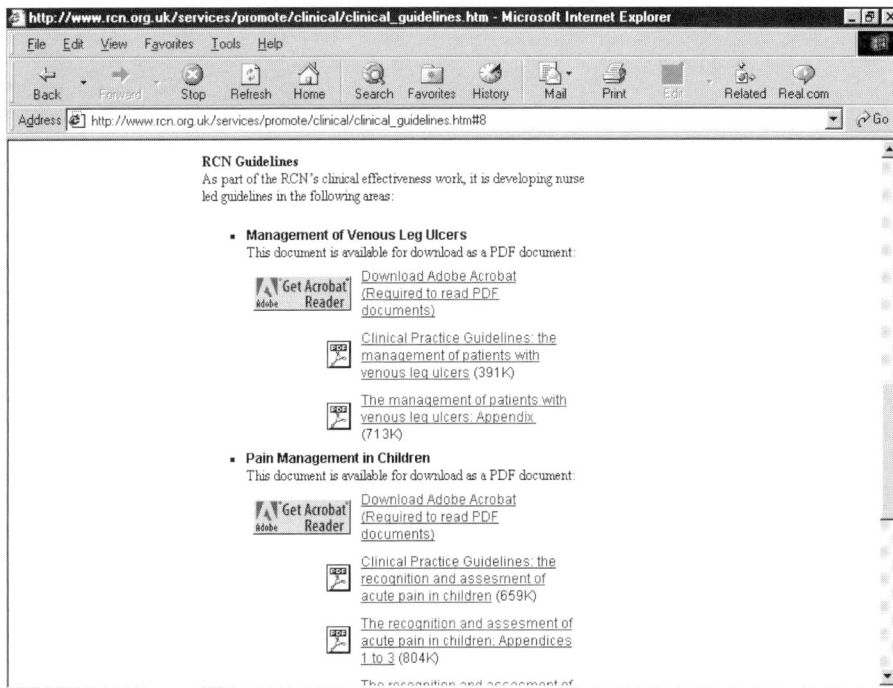

**Fig. 9.1** Nursing guidelines developed by the Royal College of Nursing

alternative and complementary pain therapies, as well as hypertext links to related Web sites.

The Royal College of Nursing, the largest professional organisation for UK nurses, has a growing site <http://www.rcn.org.uk> (Fig. 9.1), providing details about its activities, and library services. The Research & Development section has its own site <http://www.man.ac.uk/rcn/> that provides useful information on current and forthcoming events, conferences and projects.

All university departments of nursing and midwifery now have Web sites. Typically, these provide prospectus-type information, though a growing number are developing distance-learning courses that are being delivered over the Web. Examples of this include the School of Postgraduate Nursing at the University of Melbourne <http://www.nursing.unimelb.edu.au/masternurse/>, who offer a Masters degree in Nursing (Fig. 9.2) and the Loyala University in Chicago who run an online course on the Nursing Care of Patients with Respiratory Problems <http://www.luc.edu/schools/nursing/grad/online/>. Nearer to home, De Montfort University are running online courses in Tissue Viability and Clinical Guidelines.

Student nurses have particular needs and sites that have been developed to address these including Brutish Nursing <http://www.brutish-nursing.com/index.html> and the Student Nurse Underground <http://www.

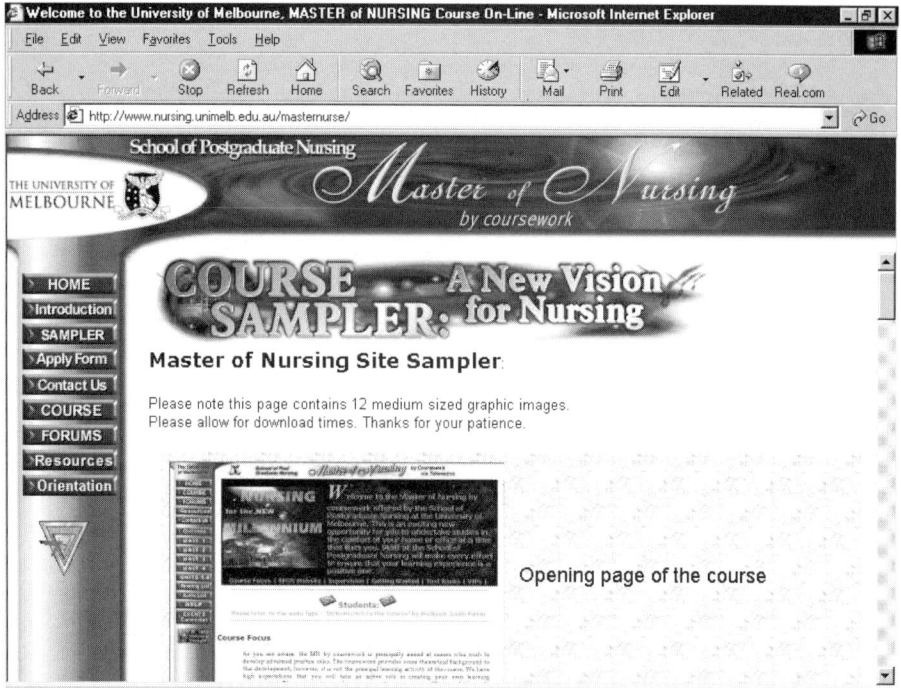

**Fig. 2** Master degree in Nursing – via the Web

coopshouse.freeserve.co.uk/> which includes a number of nursing essays on a range of topics that have previously been submitted as course-work (Fig. 9.3). Indeed, some of these essays even include details of the mark the student received!

The quality of the information on sites related to nursing and health care is an important issue, and various codes and criteria have been developed to help users develop confidence in the quality of the information. Much of the information on the Web has not been through the editorial review process and, therefore, care should be taken before basing practice on information gained in this way. A recent article by Murray and Rizzollo[1] gives a good overview of these issues.

## Mailing lists

Although Web sites are a good source of information, they do not readily enable practitioners to ask a question or create a debate with professional colleagues. To facilitate this, we must use other Internet services such as mailing lists and newsgroups.

The number of mailing lists relevant to nursing has also increased dramatically over the last few years. The biggest and most active is NurseNet[2] which, at times, distributes 50 messages a day on a wide range of topics. Other

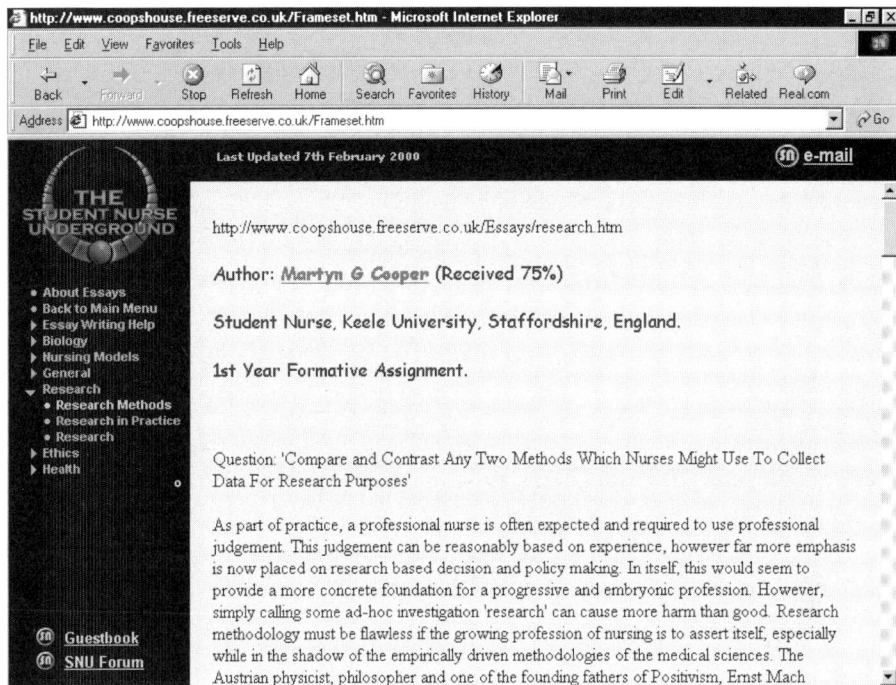

**Fig. 9.3** Online essays at the Student Nurse Underground site

lists, however, are more specific. For example, the list NurseRes[3] was established to discuss matters relating to research questions and methodology, whilst the focus of NursingEd[4] is nurse education. Smaller, less active lists have been set up for particular countries – Nurse-UK[5] is for nurses working in the UK – and for individual specialities, such as psychiatric nursing[6].

Each list has its own etiquette (or 'netiquette') and regular contributors. It is worth reading the messages for a few days before contributing yourself to ensure that you do not ask inappropriate questions.

The nursing lists are generally very supportive and posting a question or scenario and asking for help or comments can contact experts in almost any areas. Several discussions have involved questions such as 'has anyone used product...?' or 'I have a patient with this problem and I don't know what to do about...'. Responses typically come back within a few hours from fellow professionals who have dealt with similar products or patient problems, and provide other insights or avenues to help care for that patient. A large and up-to-date list of mailing lists is available from the Nursing and Health Care Resources on the Net site <http://www.shef.ac.uk/~nhcon>.

# Newsgroups

Though similar to mailing lists, Internet newsgroups do not require readers to 'subscribe' and messages do not clutter up your electronic mailbox. (Newsgroup messages are read using dedicated news reader software or via your Web browser.)

The main nursing newsgroup is <<u>sci.med.nursing</u>>, and its UK variant <<u>uk.sci.med.nursing</u>>. Postings range from 'requests for information' through to more topical debates such as staffing patterns and nursing pay. For students the premier newsgroups are <<u>bit.listserv.snurse-l</u>> and <<u>alt.support.student-nurse</u>>.

As newsgroups attract an international audience, they can be a truly useful source of information and contacts. It is worth remembering, however, that anyone can read messages sent to a newsgroup and unless the group is moderated, anyone can post messages.

# Chat rooms

An increasing number of nurses are participating in synchronous communication by the use of chat rooms, and a number of nursing-related chat rooms have been set up at the Virtual Nurse <<u>http://www.virtualnurse.com/</u>> and Cyber Nurse <<u>http://www.cyber-nurse.com/veetac/chatrooms.htm</u>>.

The conversation in these rooms can be very wide-ranging and, if the rooms are busy with lots of participants from all over the world, communication can become very rapid and occasionally confusing. Some of the chat rooms have specific times when a particular expert or well-known nursing personality will be online. At other times, there is no knowing who will be in the room, and the 'conversations' tend to be social rather than professional.

# Conclusions

The Internet provides a massive resource for nurses who require information to help them deliver patient care more effectively. In addition to this, the Internet can also help with continuing education in the form of online courses. Such courses provide an alternative to attendance at an educational institution – a factor that may suit the learning needs and commitments of many nurses. Furthermore, access to nursing literature and online forums on a 24-hour basis ensure that professional interests can be pursued at a time convenient to the nurse, rather than the local health sciences librarian.

In recognition of the growing importance of the Internet – and the need for nursing professionals to be able to readily identify high quality Internet sites, the UK higher education Joint Information Systems Committee (JISC) has recently agreed to fund the development of the Nursing, Midwives and Allied Health

Professionals (NMAHP) database <http://nmahp.ac.uk>. When launched, (scheduled for 2001) this database will provide a one-stop source for high quality Internet resources for nurses.

The Internet, however, is not a panacea – it will not meet everyone's needs all of the time. Moreover, to realise the potential of the Internet, nursing staff must invest time learning how to search for information and, more importantly, learn how to assess the information they find. Once these skills are acquired though, the potential of the Internet for nursing staff can begin to be realised.

### References

1  Murray P, Rizzollo MA. Web site reviews and evaluations *Nursing Standard On-line* <http://www.nursing-standard.co.uk/archives/vol11-45/ol-art.htm>
2  NurseNet. To subscribe, send e-mail to listserv@listserv.utoronto.ca with the message: Sub NurseNet [Your real name]
3  NurseRes. To subscribe, send e-mail to listserv@listserv.kent.edu with the message: Subscribe NurseRES [Your real name]
4  NursingEd. To subscribe, send e-mail to listserv@ulkyvm.louisville.edu with the message: Subscribe NursingEd [Your real name]
5  Nurse-UK. To subscribe send e-mail to jiscmail@jiscmail.ac.uk with the message: Join Nurse-UK [Your real name] or visit <http://www.jiscmail.ac.uk/lists/nurse-uk.html>
6  Psychiatric-Nursing. To subscribe send e-mail to jiscmail@jiscmail.ac.uk with the message: Join Psychiatric-Nursing [Your real name] or visit: <http://www.jiscmail.ac.uk/lists/psychiatric-nursing.html>

# 10

# Orthopaedic information on the Internet

Myles Clough

*Consultant Orthopaedic Surgeon at Kamloops, BC, Canada*

cloughs@wkpowerlink.com

## Introduction

Orthopaedic surgery is both well represented and well organised on the Internet. This situation is a result of there being a very early movement towards comprehensive indexing, a strong mailing list, Orthopod, <http://www.orthogate.com/mailing%20list%20stuff/index.html> and a will to cooperate. Orthopaedic surgeons recognised early on that the field was huge and that some degree of organisation, to divide up the areas of interest, would avoid wasting the rarest resource, Internet-competent orthogeeks. Orthopaedic surgery now leads all medical fields in the development of a comprehensive gateway resource, Orthogate <http://www.orthogate.com>.

## Orthopaedic sites for the specialist

The hot spots on the Internet correspond well to the hottest areas of development in the subject. Sports medicine, for example, is extremely well represented on the Internet with the sites managed by Don Johnson in Ottawa. The Practical Arthroscopy site <http://www.newsltr.com/arthro/welcome.html> is a Web version of a newsletter sent out to people with a special interest in sports medicine, whilst the Carleton Sports Medicine Clinic <http://www.carletonsportsmed.com/front.htm> is a more conventional site show-casing the clinic. What is not typical is the wealth of evaluation and surgical tips at this site. The Physician Education category, for example, provides information on topics such as 'gender issues in ACL injuries', 'groin pain in soccer players' and 'chronic Achilles tendinitis'.

69

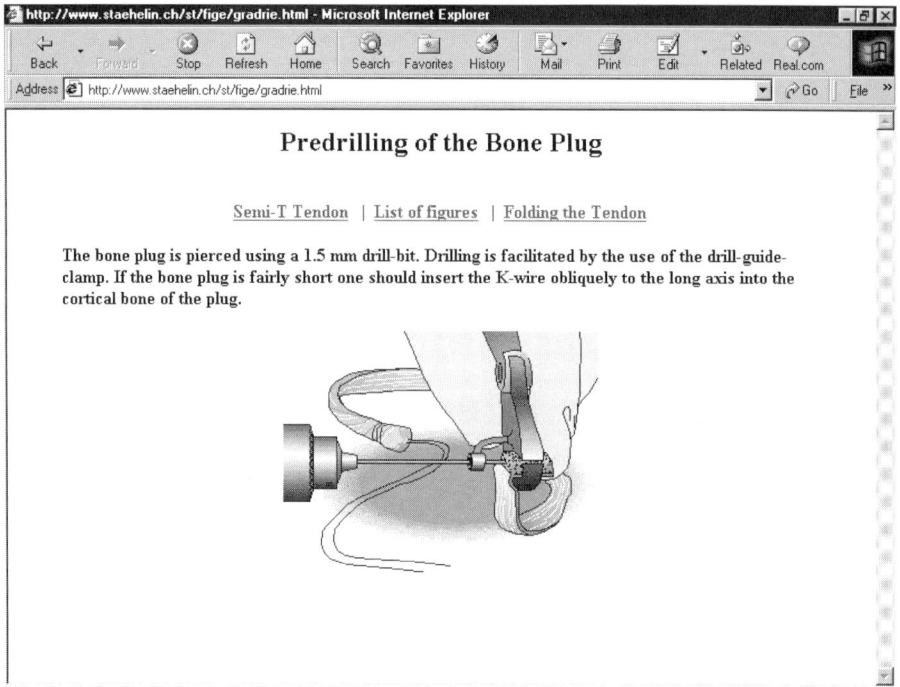

**Fig. 10.1** ACL restoration – step-by-step instructions

One of the best step-by-step descriptions of cruciate ligament operative techniques can be found at Kruzlifix's Anterior Cruciate Ligament site <http://www.staehelin.ch/index.html>. Developed by Andreas Staehelin in Switzerland, this site provides detailed information (in both a textual and graphical format) on ACL and PCL restoration using patellar tendon and semitendinosus tendon techniques (Fig. 10.1).

Hand surgery is also well represented on the Web. One of the best places to start finding information on this subject is via the e-Hand Electronic Textbook of Hand Surgery <http://www.eatonhand.com> and its classification home page <http://www.eatonhand.com/clf/clf000.htm>. From this page you can link to numerous hand-related topics, many of which are supported by high quality images.

Another interesting resource for specialists in hand surgery is the Case of the Week Collection <http://www.eatonhand.com/handbase/images.htm> derived from the Orthogate discussion list, Hand <http://www.jiscmail.ac.uk/lists/hand.html>. Each case is presented with a brief history and a collection of images and X-rays. If the topic is of particular interest, there is an option to run a pre-prepared MEDLINE search on that topic.

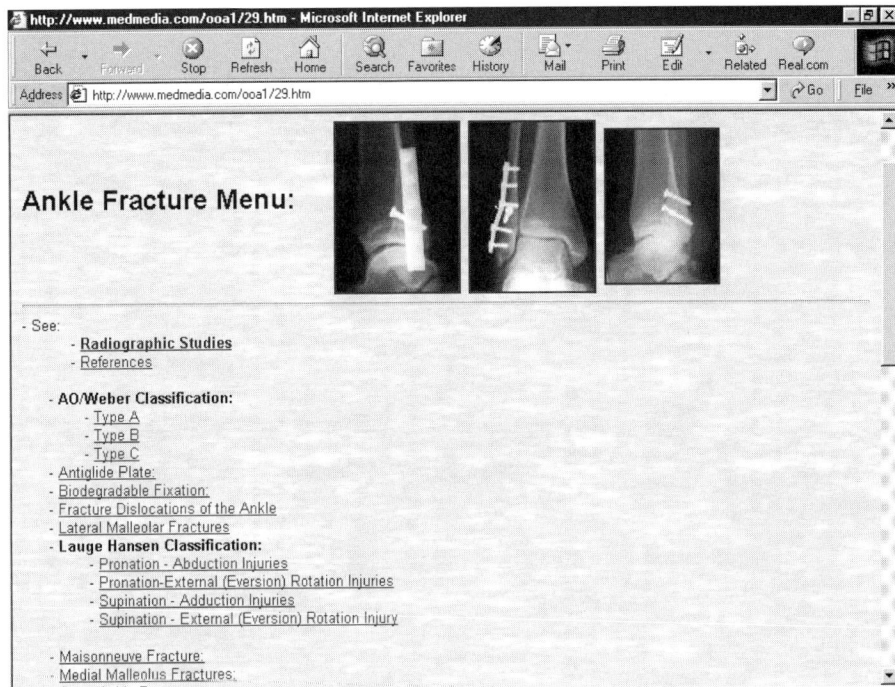

**Fig. 10.2** Wheeless' Textbook of Orthopaedics

## Orthopaedic CME sites

The premier reference site in orthopaedics, and probably the finest medical example of the use of hypertext for reference and education, is Wheeless' *Textbook of Orthopaedics* <http://www.medmedia.com> (Fig. 10.2). All the educational material Clifford Wheeless was exposed to as a resident has been collected and made into linked hypertext pages. There are now several thousand pages and over 250 megabytes of information on the site, much of it in the form of illustration. The subjects are covered in note form, for the most part, but the depth and breadth of the coverage is remarkable and the author is committed to continuously improving the material with input from contributors all over the world.

World Ortho <http://www.worldortho.com> is another gigantic achievement with its educational offerings spread more widely. Much of it is the work of Professor Huckstep from Nepean, NSW, Australia, whose textbooks and slide collection form the backbone of the site. As a site to browse, it is both educational and entertaining and it is also available as a CD-ROM for people who cannot be on-line all the time.

The Dupont Institute at the University of Delaware is another useful site with more than 60 case presentations in paediatric orthopaedics <http://gait.aidi.udel.edu/res695/homepage/pd_ortho/educate/clincase/clcasehp.htm>. Each case, prepared by a

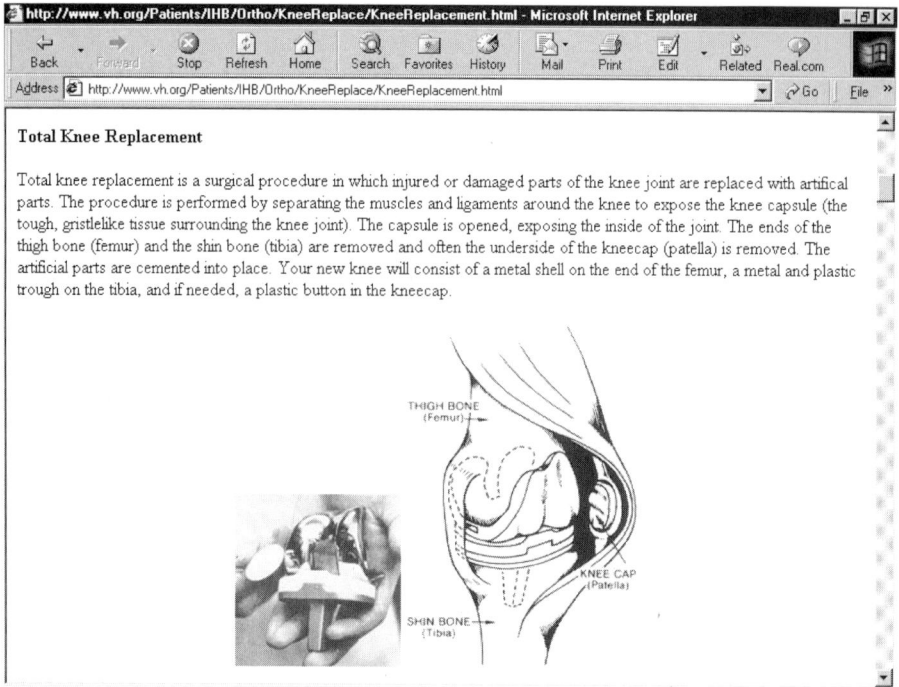

**Fig. 10.3** Patient Information from the Virtual Hospital

resident with the supervision of a staff member, is extensively illustrated and comes complete with an up-to-date bibliography. A similar effort resulted in the South Australian Orthopaedic Registrar's Notebook <http://wwwsom.fmc.flinders.edu.au/fusa/orthoweb/notebook/home.html> with topics from every area of orthopaedics. Indeed, when one considers how many careful works of scholarship are presented to critical audiences each week in teaching rounds, it is disappointing that there are not more sites doing this.

## Orthopaedics – for consumers

In the US, the medical Internet is largely seen as a way to attract patients to the institutes supporting the Web page. As a consequence of this, a great deal of effort has gone into patient information pages, many of which offer the overt message that 'the surgery is done best at our institute'. The leaders among those that do **not** do this are the American Academy of Orthopaedic Surgeons <http://www.aaos.org>, the Virtual Hospital Orthopaedic Patient Information site <http://www.vh.org/Patients/IHB/Ortho/Ortho.html> (Fig. 10.3) and the Medical Multimedia Group (MMG) <http://patient.orthogate.org>.

Among the 'come hither' group, the Southern California Orthopaedic Institute <http://www.scoi.com> does such an excellent job that their pages are now franchised to a number of other orthopaedic clinics' Web pages.

Orthopaedics is close to unique in having a group of individuals determined to combine and organise all the most useful independent orthopaedic sites into a gateway from which all the resources of the orthopaedic Internet can be reached with a few mouse-clicks. Although this aim is far from being completely realised, Orthogate <http://www.orthogate.com> is already well in advance of all other gateway sites in orthopaedics. The Orthopaedic Web Links (OWL) collection of links <http://owl.orthogate.com> is over 3000 strong and is organised into a browseable collection of pages and a searchable database. The orthopaedic-specific search engine Orthosearch <http://www.orthosearch.com>, but part of the Orthogate Project, is becoming closely integrated with the OWL database of orthopaedic sites.

Orthoguide <http://www.orthoguide.com> offers 'timesaving MEDLINE and Internet searching for orthopaedic information'. The MEDLINE option is configured to limit a search to orthopaedic and related journals, whilst the option to search the Internet is pre-configured so that only those sites identified by Othoguide as credible are searched.

There are other sites offering orthopaedic links, with the Karolinska Institute <http://www.mic.ki.se/Diseases/c5.html> prominent among them.

OMNI <http://omni.ac.uk> also has a list of high quality sites, though the number of orthopaedic links is relatively small. Typically, the 'megasites' which try to offer a gateway to the whole of the medical Internet offer collections of orthopaedic pages numbering about 100 or less. OWL/Orthogate currently has links to more than 3000 pages, and perhaps more importantly, the collection is complied by orthopaedic surgeons with a view to selecting sites which we think would interest other orthopaedic surgeons.

## The future

No one who has used the Internet for serious scholarship can doubt that academic research and communication will, in the future, be conducted largely on the Internet. The low cost, the ease of searching, the nearly instant availability, and the use of hypertext links for illustrating and cross-referencing, together make a compelling case. It is not a question of **if** this transformation will occur but **when**. In orthopaedics, we believe strongly that it will be soon and we are prepared to propel our subject rapidly in that direction. When it does occur there will be a central portal which will direct readers to resources and comment on the quality of the content. Such portals will be necessary in all subjects to reduce the information overload, so graphically described as 'drinking from a firehose'.[1] We recommend that all medical and surgical specialties come to grips with this likely future and determine how they would like the gateway in their subject to arise. There are a number of commercial sites and medical libraries who are working hard to occupy this position. In orthopaedics, we have made a clear statement that we want the gateway to be run by orthopaedists, for orthopaedists.

### References

1  Waldrop MM. Learning to drink from a fire hose. *Science* 1990; **248**: 674–5

# 11

# Pharmacy resources on the Internet

Michelle Wake* and Linda Lisgarten†

*Deputy Librarian, The School of Pharmacy,
University of London, UK
†Librarian and Head of Information Services, The School of Pharmacy,
University of London, UK

library@ulsop.ac.uk

## Introduction

At the present time the role the Internet plays in providing drug information is under great scrutiny. In the main, this debate centres on whether or not the UK ban on the advertising of licensed prescription drugs to the general public can continue in the face of the global nature of the Internet. This problem is exacerbated by the fact that providing factual information about prescription medicines – 'authorised by competent authorities' – is allowed in the European Union[1]. Differing national laws regarding the sales of medicines direct to the general public further complicate this issue. In The Netherlands, for example, patients can buy drugs by mail order[2], whilst in the US there are on-line pharmacies that have been known to supply patients with any medicine without a prescription[3].

The breaking down of national borders has other implications for those who seek drug information as drug names, generic as well as proprietary, can vary from country to country. For example, paracetamol is referred to as acetaminophen in the US. Moreover, what is licensed for use in one country might not be in another. Arguably the most highly publicised example of this was sildenafil (Viagra) which was licensed in the US some 6 months earlier than in the UK[4].

Despite very valid concerns regarding the quality of information on the Internet and whether the Internet is an appropriate medium for selling medicines, there is a great deal of useful pharmaceutical material available on the Internet for all levels of user[5]. This chapter highlights some of the most useful pharmacy resources on the Internet trying, where possible, to highlight UK resources.

## Pharmacy directories

The first structured pharmaceutical information server was PharmWeb <http://www.pharmweb.net>, established in 1994 by Dr AJ D'Emanuele at the University of Manchester. It not only indexes Web pages, but also creates and manages Web sites for a range of organisations. It is designed mainly for professionals, with directories of newsgroups, mailing lists, companies, societies, government bodies, conferences and a list of vacancies. There are also lists of pharmacy schools and information on educational resources. Although based in the UK, it is mirrored in six countries and deals with information from around the globe.

The London and South Eastern Drug Information Service provides DrugInfoZone <http://www.druginfozone.org>, another service aimed at health professionals. It has a useful drug news section, full-text of recent issues of current awareness bulletins and provides monthly bibliographic citations (derived from the PharmLine database) on 44 key topics.

Most pharmacy gateways are from the US, but one that has a UK mirror and lists UK resources, is the Virtual Library Pharmacy section <http://www.cpb.uokhsc.edu/pharmacy/pharmint.html>. Note, however, that the list of government Web servers in this directory makes no mention of the NHS!

The US marketing company Mediconsult.com manages the Pharmaceutical Information Network, PharmInfo <http://www.pharminfo.com>. This service provides brief descriptions of a number of resources and has a drug database (DrugDB) that links to a number of full-text resources. This database can also be browsed using generic and/or trade names, though the US focus of this product means it has to be used with care in the UK.

There are two major UK gateways for those interested in the pharmaceutical industry, PharmiWeb and InPharm. PharmiWeb <http://www.pharmiweb.com> provides news, employment opportunities and company information, whilst InPharm.com <http://www.inpharm.com> has been set up to demonstrate to pharmaceutical and health care executives what the Internet can provide and thus encourage the creation of commercial sites. InPhram includes directories of organisations, companies and freelancers in medical communications as well as vacancies and industry news. The site also publishes regular Internet 'tours' that highlight sites relevant to a specific subject. Subjects covered recently include alcoholism, genomics and R&D advances.

At present, most UK government and society sites only provide details of their roles, structure and coming events. They do not, as yet, provide indexes of drugs. Government bodies include the Medicines Control Agency <http://www.open.gov.uk/mca/mcahome.htm>, the Committee on the Safety of Medicines <http://www.open.gov.uk/mca/csmhome.htm> and the Prescription Pricing Authority <http://www.ppa.org.uk>.

The professional and governing body for UK pharmacy is the Royal Pharmaceutical Society of Great Britain. Its Web site <http://www.rpsgb.org.uk> has a news section and useful list of links.

The Association of the British Pharmaceutical Industry (ABPI) at <http://www.abpi.org.uk> provides a site that lists all its members, around a hundred companies producing prescription medicines in the UK and links to their Web sites where available. Publications published by the Association include booklets concerned with treatments for specific conditions. Although it is not possible to view the full text of these documents, ordering information is given.

Finally, both the United Kingdom Drug Information Pharmacists Group <http://www.ukdipg.org.uk> and the Association of Information Officers in the Pharmaceutical Industry <http://www.aiopi.org.uk> have lists of useful links.

## Journals and books

The most recent issues of the *Pharmaceutical Journal* are available in full-text, without charge, at <http://www.pharmj.com>. All of the classified advertisements – which include employment vacancies – can be searched by job function and/or geographical area. As the official journal of the Royal Pharmaceutical Society of Great Britain, this is a valuable resource with news, views and original research papers.

For details of other on-line pharmacy journals the Virtual Pharmacy Library and PharmWeb, discussed above, are highly recommended. The Virtual Pharmacy, for example, currently provides links to over 50 specialised pharmacy titles.

Another rich source of information is the Electronic Medicines Compendium <http://www.emc.vhn.net> (Fig. 11.1). This resource contains all the information that is included in the *ABPI Compendium of Data Sheets* and *Summaries of Product Characteristics*. In total, this compendium contains details of more than 2500 medicines licensed in the UK. Searching by both the generic and product name is supported. The site is divided into professional, general public and industry sections for which registration (no fee) is required.

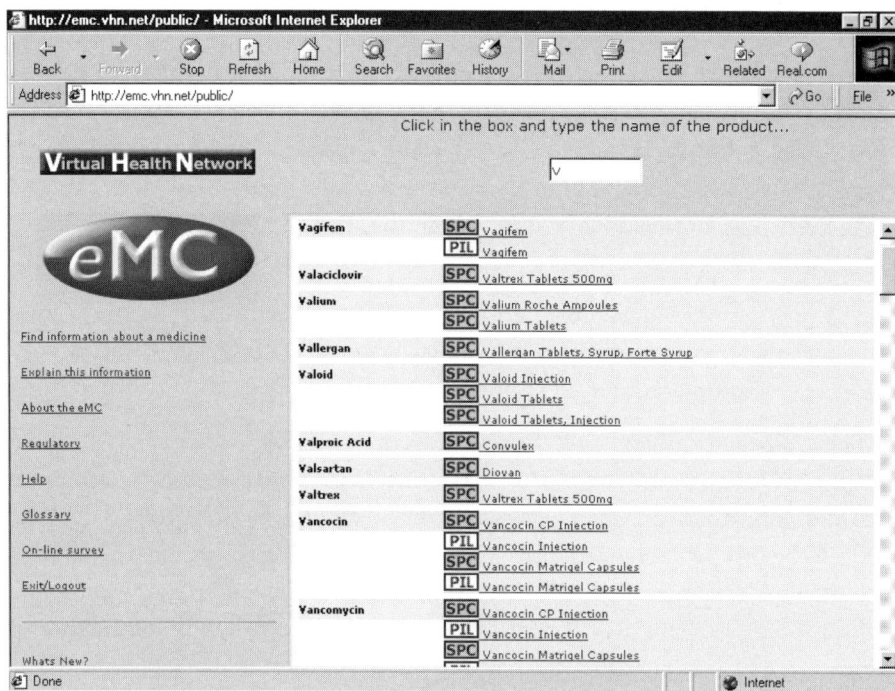

**Fig. 11.1** ABPI compendium of data sheets.

The British National Formulary <http://www.bnf.org>, which provides up-to-date information designed for health care professionals on prescribing, dispensing and administration of medicines, was launched onto the Web in 2000. Published twice a year by the British Medical Association and the Royal Pharmaceutical Society of Great Britain, the Web version will be issued simultaneously with the printed version, but will include extra sections, such as news, which can be up-dated regularly. The BNF can be searched as well as browsed (Fig. 11.2).

The UK Pharmacopoeia also has a Web site <http://www.pharmacopoeia.org.uk/>, but access to the monographs is restricted to subscribers to the printed or CD-ROM Pharmacopoeia products.

## Patient information

Drug information aimed specifically for UK patients is thin on the ground, especially when compared to what is available in the US. The Electronic Medicines Compendium (discussed above) is certainly the most comprehensive source.

Patient UK <http://www.patient.co.uk>, set up by two GPs in Newcastle, has a Medicines and Drugs section <http://www.patient.co.uk/drugs.htm>, which helpfully provides a list of UK Web sites. There is also a directory of non-UK

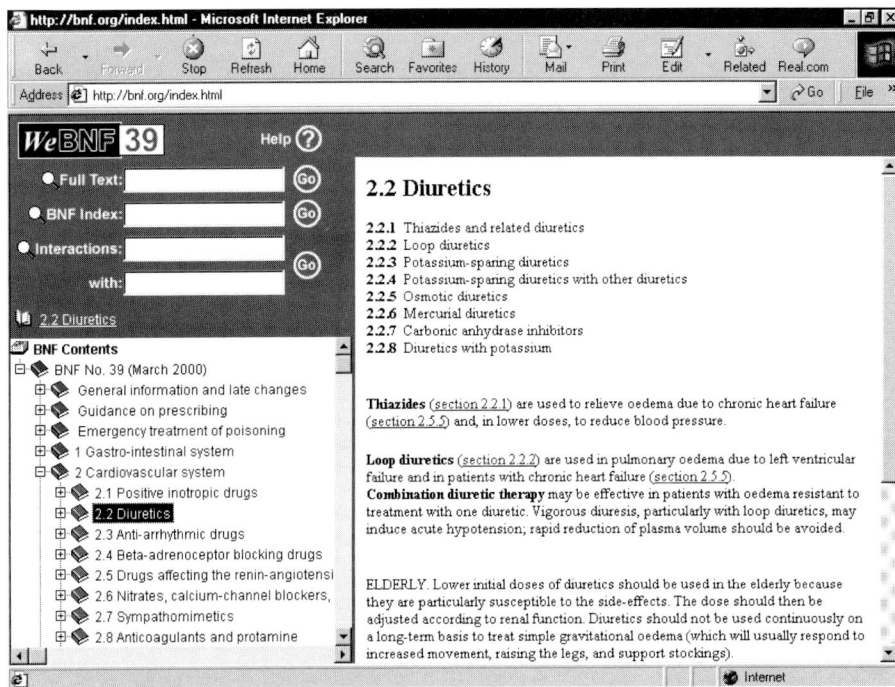

**Fig. 11.2** The electronic BNF – both searchable and browseable.

sites but the authors highlight the problems UK patients may experience in using these resources.

The National Pharmaceutical Association has an 'Ask Your Pharmacist Site' <http://www.askyourpharmacist.co.uk> which provides a directory of pharmacies and has a page of basic information on choosing, using and storing medicines. Unusually, this site has a children's page, with cartoon pictures than can be printed out and coloured in, which emphasises important facts about medicines.

PharmWeb also has a section for patients. This gives information on topics such as how to use medicines and how to treat common ailments such as coughs and colds. Though these pages are still 'under development' what is available is both good and authoritative.

Perhaps one of the best sites for patients is InteliHealth <http://www.intelihealth.com> produced by the Harvard Medical School and Aetna US Healthcare. At this site, information about drugs can be found by using brand or generic names. It is also possible to browse medication specific to certain conditions. Once a drug has been identified, a link is provided to the US Pharmacopoeia database where additional information – such as adverse effects, contra-indications, etc. – can be found. There is also a section on new drugs

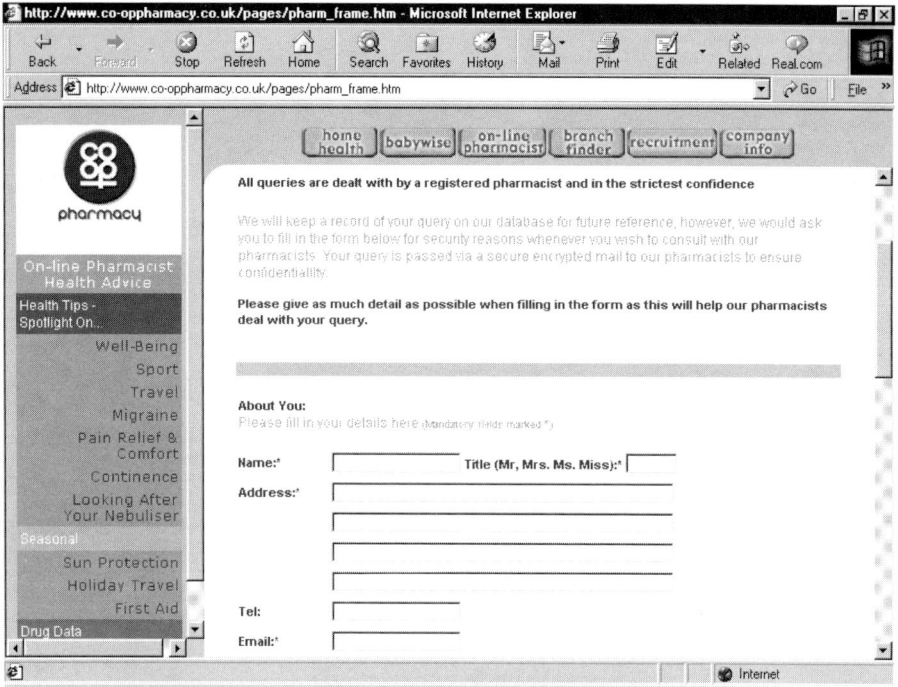

**Fig. 11.3** Registered pharm,acists reader to answer your queriues.

recently approved by the US Food and Drug Administration and a news section that details warnings and recalls by the FDA. Although InteliHealth aims to 'consumerise' health information, there is much of interest to the professional on this site including a 'Professional Network' section. The FDA's own Web site <http://www.fda.gov> has patient as well as professional sections.

Similarly, PharmInfo has a large section aimed at patients. The 'Disease Center' section, for example, <http://www.pharminfo.com/disease/disdb_mnu.html> provides links organised by disease. These links provide general information, drug information, news, articles and lists of other relevant sources. Inevitably there is a strong US bias. No UK patient support groups, for example, were listed under Breast Cancer.

Finally, patients can now obtain free on-line pharmacy consultations over the Web. The National Co-operative Pharmacy site <http://www.co-oppharmacy.co.uk> undertakes to answer any health-related query within two working days. All questions are answered by qualified pharmacists (Fig. 11.3).

## Discussion lists and newsgroups

One of the longest running pharmacy discussion lists is the Pharmacy Mail Exchange <http://www.dmu.ac.uk/ln/pme> at De Montfort University. This list is moderated and only open to pharmacists and health care professionals. Another restricted-access list is the Private-Rx service <http://www.private-rx.net>. This service provides various discussion lists for UK registered pharmacists.

For a more general discussion about issues relevant to pharmacy, the Usenet newsgroup <news://uk.sci.med.pharmacy> is worth consulting. Not only is this resource open to everyone, but the archive of previous postings can be found online at <http://www.deja.com/group/uk.sci.med.pharmacy>.

An exhaustive list of other pharmacy related newsgroups and discussion lists can be found on the PharmWeb server.

## Conclusions

There is much for pharmaceutical professionals and their patients to gain from the Internet in terms of information retrieval and dissemination. The debate as to whether or not UK pharmacists should provide services over the Internet has stepped up a gear in recent times. In September 1999 when the UK's first Internet pharmacy opened for business <http://www.pharmacy2u.co.uk>. Following this, in January 2000, the Council of the Royal Pharmaceutical Society of Great Britain announced standards for pharmacists providing services over the Internet[6].

Although the Internet cannot replace the patient–pharmacist relationship, it can complement it and can be used to encourage greater contact with the general public[7]. Already, an increasing number of pharmaceutical professionals have been developing high quality Web sites and undertaking training to help realise this goal[8].

### References

1   Anon. Medicines information allowed on the Internet. *Pharm J* 1999; **262**: 828

2   Anon. Selling medicines via the Internet. *Pharm J* 1999; **263**: 720

3   Anon. US move to regulate Internet prescription medicine sales. *Pharm J* 2000; **264**: 85

4   Anon. The challenge of the Internet. *Pharm J* 1998; **261**: 867

5   Eysenbach G, Diepgen TL. Towards quality management of medical information on the Internet evaluation, labelling, and filtering of information. *BMJ* 1998; **317**: 1496–500 <http://www.bmj.com/cgi/content/full/317/7171/1496> [Accessed 30 August 2000]

6   Anon. Council sets standards for Internet pharmacy. *Pharm J* 2000; **264**: 9

7   Widman L, Tong D. Requests for medical advice from patients and families to health care providers who publish on the World Wide Web. *Arch Intern Med* 1997; **157**: 209–12 <http://www.bmj.com/cgi/content/full/317/7171/1496> [Accessed 30 August 2000]

8   Anon. Psychiatric pharmacy Internet project. *Pharm J* 1999; **262**: 826

# 12

# Professional health portals in the UK

Robert Kiley

*Head of Systems Strategy – Wellcome Library for the History &
Understanding of Medicine, London, UK*

r.kiley@wellcome.ac.uk

## Introduction

The development of information portals for UK health professionals has stepped up a gear. The past few months, for example, have witnessed the launch of services such as Physicians-Decisions <http://www.pdxmd.com>, MedicDirect <http://www.medicdirect.co.uk>, Medix-UK <http://www.medix-uk.com> and DoctorsWorld <http://www.doctorsworld.com>. These new services join the more established ones such as Doctors.Net <http://www.doctors.net.uk>, Medic8 <http://www.medic8.com> and NetDoctorPro <http://www.netdoctorpro.co.uk>. Even these portals are relatively new, however, when compared with some of the more established US services such as Medscape <http://www.medscape.com> and WebMD <http://www.webmd.com>. Although the total number of professional portals is difficult to calculate, a search on the Health on the Net database suggests that there are more than 300.

Which of these portals offer the best services and are worth registering with? Some simply provide access to publicly available databases like MEDLINE, whilst others allow their members to access value-added services such as subscription-based databases, full-text journals and online textbooks. This article will look at a number of the leading medical portals and highlight what services they offer. Health professionals can use this guide to pick the portal that addresses their needs most closely.

# Selection criteria

In deciding which portals to look at I devised the following simple criteria:

- *The portals must provide a doctors-only service (accessible via a registration);*
- *The service should be aimed at UK health professionals;*
- *The site must be indexed by either OMNI, or Health on the Net;*
- *An AltaVista 'link' search should identify at least 10 other Internet sites that link to that site.*

Using these criteria the following portals, in alphabetical order, were selected for analysis: Doctors.net; MedicDirect; NetDoctorPro and UKPractice.net

## Doctors.net

**Address**
<http://www.doctors.net.uk> (Fig. 12.1).

**Registration**
Online form. GMC number required. No fee.

**Owners/Partners**
Independent peer-led Internet resource for the UK medical profession. Ethical and Editorial Committee includes representatives from medical schools, post-graduate deans and professional bodies.

**Analysis**
With some 40,000 members – approximately 35% of all practising doctors in the UK – Doctors.Net is able to offer information-providers an easy and cost-effective way of distributing information to doctors. For example, clinical guidelines from the National Institute of Clinical Evidence (NICE), and new reports and recommendations from the Medical Devices Agency (MDA) and the Committee for the Safety of Medicines (CSM) are distributed, on publication, to all members of this portal.

Members also get access to the full version of the Cochrane Library (all six databases, including the Database of Systematic Reviews, DARE and NEED) and to a number of online medical textbooks including *Harrison's Principles of Internal Medicine*, Marshall's *Clinical Biochemistry* and Kumar and Clark's *Clinical Medicine*.

The site also provides access to MEDLINE and a highly useful facility called JournAlert. This allows users to save a MEDLINE search and receive email updates when any new articles, relevant to that search, are indexed by this database. Numerous other services are available including discussion forums, online presentations, and a database of current vacancies. Doctors.net recently launched WirelessMed, the first WAP service for the medical industry to provide doctors with rapid access to vital information when they are away from the surgery or hospital.

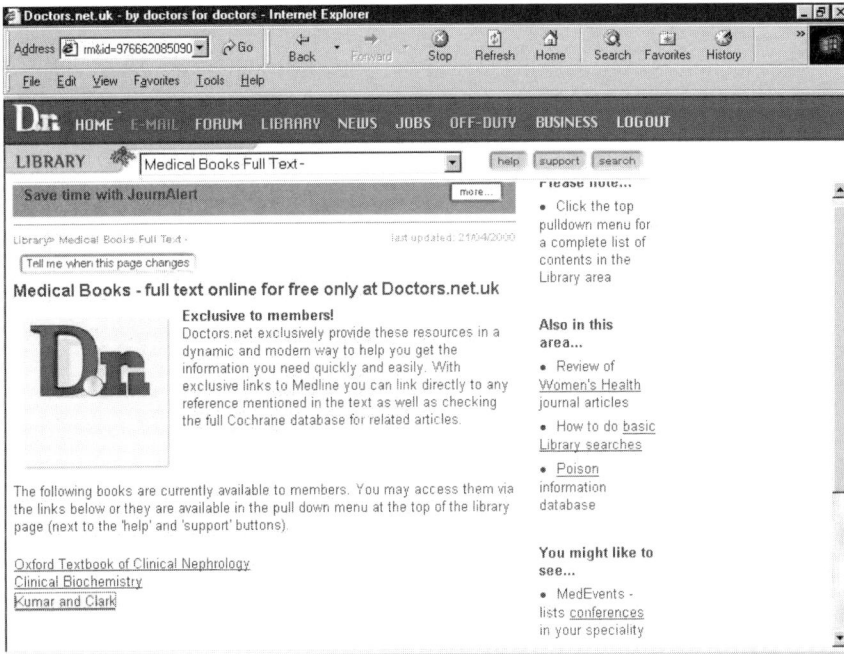

**Fig. 12.1** Doctorsnet is an independent peer-led Internet resource for the UK medical profession

Registered users are also provided with a Web-enabled email account – ensuring mail can be picked up irrespective of where the doctor is located – and a customised view of the service and the content available based upon the users' specialty.

## MedicDirect

**Address**
<http://www.dr.medicdirect.co.uk/> (Fig. 12.2).

**Registration**
Online form. GMC number required. No fee.

**Owners/Partners**
Independent site developed by a number of UK medical consultants, including three professors and fifteen honorary senior lecturers. Details of the specialists responsible for this service are available at the MedicDirect site.

**Analysis**
An information-rich portal that provides registered users with a range of unique resources including a searchable slide library with over 1200 downloadable images, online lectures, and around 40 video and audio clips highlighting key practical procedures such as the Heimlich manoeuvre and lumbar puncture.

Guide to Healthcare Resources on the Internet

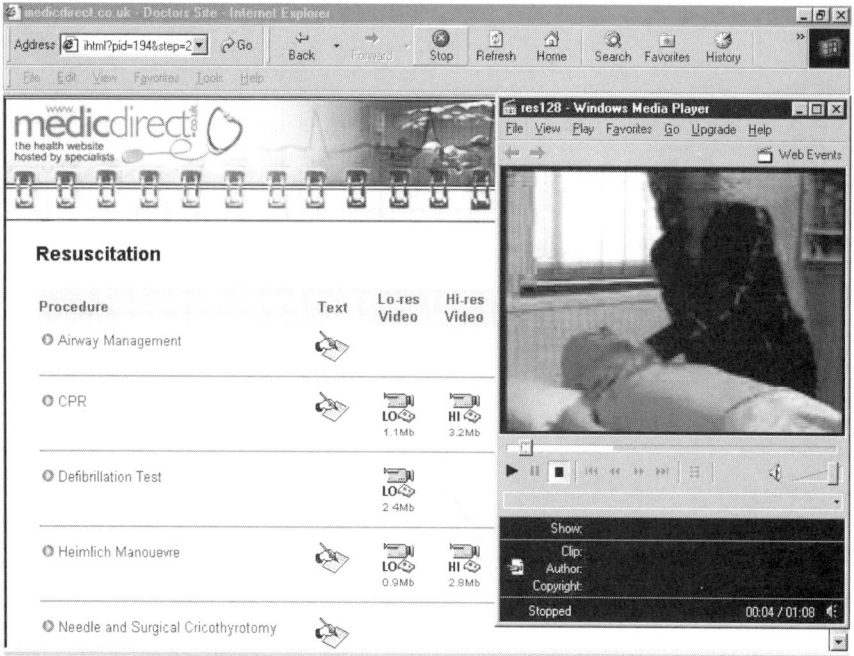

**Fig. 12.2** MedicDirect is an independent site developed by a number of UK medical consultants, including three professors and fifteen honorary senior lecturers.

Registered users can also get exclusive online access to the *Prescribers' Journal*, which deals with the latest therapeutic advances in drug treatment. Online calculators (burns, body mass index etc) and scoring protocols such as the Cage Score (for determining alcoholic risk) and the Barthel Activity of Daily Living are also available in an easy to use Web-format.

The site also has information on forthcoming courses, current vacancies, and various discussion forums, whilst the online library provides the usual access to MEDLINE and links to over 1000 journals, searchable by specialty. Note, however, that MedicDirect simply directs you to the relevant journal's home page. Whether or not the full-text of that journal is available is dependent upon the publisher.

Users can also get access to a range of patient information sheets, presented in a pdf format for easy printing and distribution. Though undoubtedly a good idea, the lack of details relating to who authored each leaflet, when it was published and last updated, undermines the usefulness of this section. The site also provides a link to Toxbase, though to get access to this poisons database you need to register directly with the database provider.

*NetDoctor.Pro*

**Address**
<http://www.netdoctorpro.co.uk/>

**Registration**
Online form. GMC number not required. No fee.

**Owners/Partners**
Netdoctor.Pro is an offshoot of the publicly accessible NetDoctor (<http://www.netdoctor.co.uk>) service. This site has been created by a number of health professionals. Details of the Medical Panel and the ethical principles the site adopts can be found online.

**Analysis**
Registered users can gain access to the full version of the Cochrane Library and Harrison's *Principles of Internal Medicine*. And, though the NetDoctor.Pro site warns users than only a limited number of members can access these resources at one time, on the occasions I used it I experienced no difficulties.

The site also provides access to a range of databases, and though all the ones listed are freely available on the Internet the team at NetDoctor have brought together, in one accessible place, a good collection of resources. This list includes all the key databases such as MEDLINE and BioethicsLine, as well as other less well known products, such as the complementary and alternative medicine database from the Office of Alternative Medicine and the Alcohol database from the National Institute on Alcohol Abuse and Alcoholism.

Users can also access an impressive looking list of online journals, all of which have been categorised by subject. However, as with the databases, users are simply pointed to the journals' publicly accessible Web site. Being a member of NetDoctor.Pro does not open any doors in terms of full-text access. Perhaps more irritating, however, was the fact that a number of links to these titles were dead.

The site also has a weekly 'Guess the diagnosis quiz'. Members who complete this correctly are entered into a prize draw.

*UKPracticeNet*

**Address**
<http://www.ukpractice.net/>

**Registration**
Online registration form. GMC number required. No fee.

**Owner/Partners**
The site has been developed with a range of partners including The Royal College of General Practitioners and the National Association of Primary Care. Other organisations with close links to this service include the Royal Marsden hospital and MIND.

Launched in September 1999 ukpractice.net provides healthcare professionals with free access to a range of online education and reference sources.

Perhaps of greatest interest are the PGEA-accredited training courses that are available free of charge to registered GPs. Courses running at the time of writing (October 2000) include Management Skills, Finance, and Health and Safety at Work as well as more clinical courses dealing with topics such as headache, melanoma and diabetes. On completion of any course a PGEA certificate is mailed to your registered address.

The site also has a number of full-text reference sources including the *Oxford Handbook of Clinical Medicine*, an interactive version of Guillebaud's text *Contraception: your questions answered* and access to the full archive of the *Education for General Practice* journal. Users can also access a range of decision-support tools that can be used to help professionals draw up clinical guidelines. Decision-support tools are currently available for five conditions, including irritable bowel syndrome, depression and hypertension.

Registered users can also access HealthIndex – a searchable database of self help groups – and GP Literature, a database containing a list of papers and reviews relevant to general practice aimed at Registrars and doctors preparing for the MRCGP. However, as this has not been updated for over 12 months its value is questionable.

Finally, the site provides visitors with access to key policy documents such as the NHS Plan and the GMC Consultation paper – *Revalidating Doctors* – plus useful quick reference guides such as the Red Book, NHS Fees and the Travel Health Guide.

## Which is the best?

Having looked in some detail at these portals it is very difficult to say which one is the best. I believe that the Doctors.net service offers the biggest range of value-added services in terms of database provision, online textbooks and alerting services. Moreover, the ability to pick up email sent to your Doctors.net account from any Internet-ready computer is another useful service offered by this portal.

If, however, you want to access online PGEA-accredited courses, or a large collection of online images and videos then both the MedicDirect and UKPractice.Net services are worth joining. Both of these portals offer services that are exclusive to their members. Even the NetDoctor.Pro service – probably the weakest of the four portals examined here – offers some useful services, including a good collection of online databases and journals and, via its online quiz, the opportunity to enter into a weekly prize draw.

As all the services described here are available without charge to UK health professionals, I would recommend that you sign-up for all four portals and use the best bits from each.

# 13

# Finding health information on the Internet

Robert Kiley

*Head of Systems Strategy – Wellcome Library for the History & Understanding of Medicine, London, UK*

r.kiley@wellcome.ac.uk

## Introduction

As a medical librarian, the question I am most frequently asked takes the form 'how can I search the Internet for information on...?'. In an attempt to answer this, this chapter will provide a template for searching the Internet. Inevitably, how far you wish to pursue a search will depend on your own needs and circumstances. For example, whereas a house officer requiring some background information on a particular subject may limit his search to some key bibliographic databases, a nurse, interested in determining how individuals cope with a particular disease, may wish to search further and examine postings made to newsgroups and discussion lists.

In this article, I will describe how key sources such as bibliographic databases and evaluated Internet subject gate-ways can be searched. I will then extend the scope of the search and examine Web search engines, newsgroups and discussion lists. Finally, I will highlight ways in which the Internet can be used to help health professionals keep abreast of new information and research. To provide a subject theme for this column, I will describe how I searched for information on managing chronic fatigue syndrome (CFS).

## Step 1 – Bibliographic databases

Perversely, one of the main problems with the Internet is that it appears very easy to search. Both Netscape and Internet Explorer have 'search buttons' that, on

**Table 13.1** Key bibliographic databases available on the Web

---

**MEDLINE** <http://www.ncbi.nlm.nih.gov/PubMed>
Over 11 million citations. Some links to full-text articles. Free of charge.

**Cochrane Reviews** <http://www.update-software.com/cochrane/cochrane-frame.html>
Best single source of reliable evidence about the effects of health care. Abstracts available without charge. Subscription required to read the full text of the reviews and protocols.

**EMBASE** <http://www.healthgate.com/embase/search-embase-pre.shtml>
6.5 million citations. Indexes more European journals than MEDLINE, and has better coverage of pharmacology resources. Free searching – charged for full citations ($2.00 per citation). Registration required.

**CINAHL** <http://www.healthgate.com/cinahl/search-cinahl-pre.shtml>
Database of nursing and allied health literature. Free searching – charged for full citations ($1.50 per citation). Registration required.

**PsycINFO** <http://www.healthgate.com/psycinfo/search-psycinfo-pre.shtml>
Key database for references in the field of psychology and psychiatry. Free searching – charged for full citations ($0.75 per citation). Registration required.

**BIOETHICSLINE** <http://igm.nlm.nih.gov/>
Dating from 1973, BIOETHICSLINE provides health professionals with a one-stop shop to the world's bioethical research literature. Free of charge.

**HealthSTAR** <http://igm.nlm.nih.gov/>
The Health Services, Technology, Administration, and Research database is particularly useful for identifying research into patient outcomes, the effectiveness of clinical procedures, and information relating to healthcare administration and planning. Free of charge.

**CancerLit** <http://cnetdb.nci.nih.gov/cancerlit.shtml>
Product of the National Cancer Institute, this database consists of 1.3 million citations, dating from 1963. Free of charge.

---

clicking, take you to a Web search engine where you are encouraged to enter you search terms. However, though keying-in the search term is easy, sifting through the numerous 'hits' is much more time consuming and problematic.

Consequently, for all medical/health information search the best place to start is with the more traditional bibliographic databases. The core medical databases are listed in Table 13.1. If, however, your subject is not answered by these resources, a listing of other bibliographic databases can be found at: <http://www.shef.ac.uk/~scharr/ir/trawling.html>.

### Search analysis

A simple search on MEDLINE for chronic fatigue syndrome (CFS) identified over 1500 references. However, by using the 'clinical queries methodology filters' and restricting the search to the study category therapy, with the emphasis on specificity, the number of hits was reduced to a more manageable 42 citations (Fig. 13.1). The Cochrane Database yielded just one protocol, on cognitive

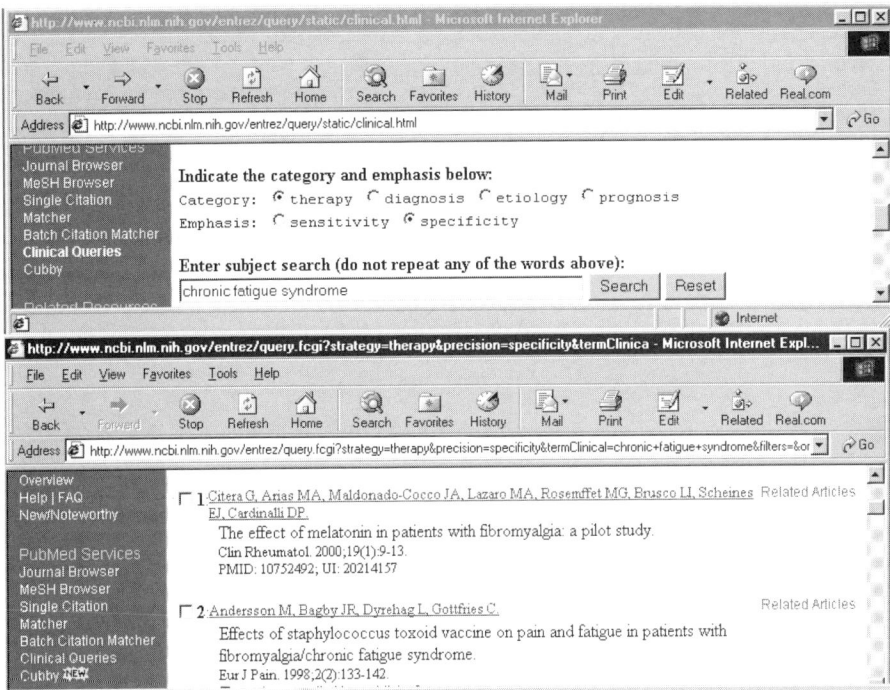

**Fig. 13.1** MEDLINE search and results using the clinical queries filter.

behaviour therapy for adults with chronic fatigue syndrome. To read this you need to set up an online subscription to the Cochrane Library (2000 price: £120.00 for one year's access).

For completeness, I also searched PsycINFO, using the strategy 'chronic fatigue syndrome AND therapy'. Limiting this to articles published in the past two years identified around 50 references. By browsing through the titles I could then select – and pay – for those references that sounded relevant and had not been picked up by my MEDLINE search.

## Step 2 – Evaluated Internet subject gateways

To extend the search and find material that has been published on the Web, it is necessary to search a number of evaluated subject gateways. As their name implies these search services provide the user with a gateway to resources on the Internet. However, rather than provide a comprehensive listing of Internet sites, only those that meet a defined quality threshold are included. Table 13.2 details a number of the premier Internet health gateways. For a more comprehensive list of evaluated gateways see <http://henry.ugl.lib.umich.edu/megasite/>.

**Table 13.2** Premier evaluated subject gateways

---

**OMNI**          <http://omni.ac.uk/>
The UK's gateway to high quality biomedical Internet resources. All resources meet the quality criterion as defined by the OMNI Advisory Group for Evaluation Criteria.

**Medical Matrix**     <http://www.medmatrix.org/>
Aimed primarily at US physicians and health workers, the Medical Matrix assigns ranks to Internet resources based on their utility for point-of-care clinical application. Quality, peer review, full content, multimedia features, and unrestricted access are emphasized in the rankings.

**MEDLINEplus**     <http://www.medlineplus.gov/>
Developed by the US National Library of Medicine, MEDLINEplus provides a gateway to high quality consumer-health resources on the Internet.

---

### Search analysis

A search of the OMNI database identified eight resources relevant to CFS, including a collection of articles published in the *British Medical Journal*[1] and a electronic discussion list, co-cure[2], that focuses on the treatment of CFS. Searching the Medical Matrix database highlights additional resources, including details of a moderated e-mail discussion list, limited to doctors and devoted to clinical concerns regarding this syndrome[3]. As none of the resources indexed by these two services was duplicated by the other, it can be inferred that, if you want a comprehensive search of the Internet, you must be prepared to search multiple gateways. The much sought after 'one-stop infomation source' has yet to appear.

Finally, to identify material that would be suitable for consumers, I searched MEDLINEplus (Fig. 13.2). Various resources were identified, including a pamphlet produced by the Centers for Disease Control and Prevention (CDC)[4] and a fact sheet authored by the National Institute of Allergy and Infectious Diseases[5].

## Step 3 – Web search engines

A joint study published by Inktomi and the NEC Research Institute in January 2000 estimated that the number of indexable pages on the Web now exceeds 1 billion[6]. (The indexable Web refers to those pages that search engines can reach. Web search engines do not index web pages that are generated on the fly – for example results from a MEDLINE search – or those that can only be accessed by password holders.) Of greater significance, however, is the fact that even the biggest search engines (Google and AltaVista) only index around 50% of the Web[7]. Consequently, if you require an exhaustive search you should not rely exclusively on one search engine.

For most users, however, the problems relating to an exhaustive search seem somewhat irrelevant when the existing search engines – whatever their limitations

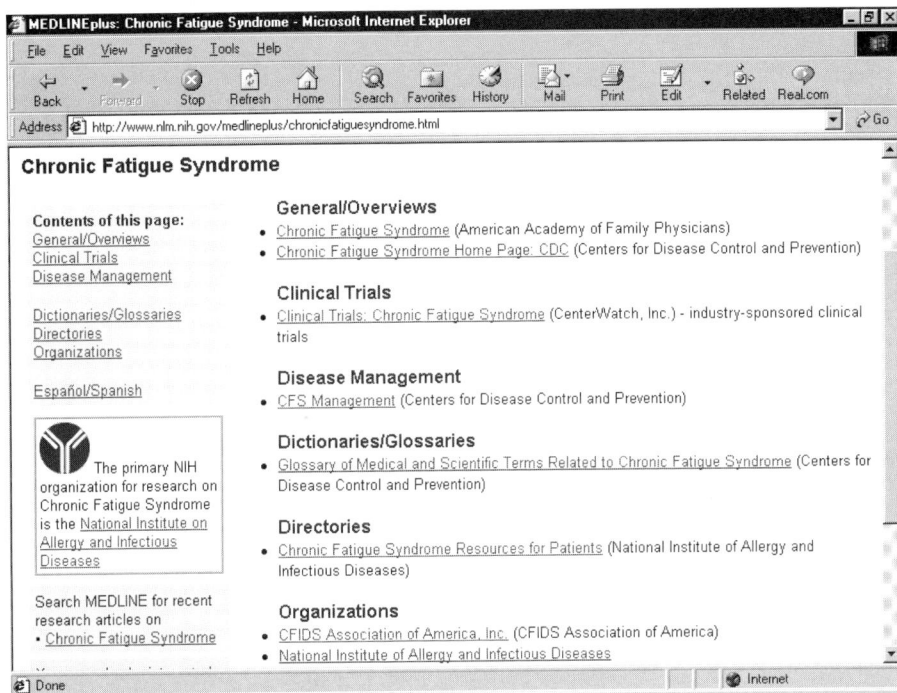

**Fig. 13.2** Evaluated patient information from MEDLINEplus.

– already identify too many pages. Indeed, a search of AltaVista for 'chronic fatigue syndrome' identifies over 18,000 Web pages. In many ways though, the large number of 'relevant' hits is a reflection of a poorly defined search strategy. As discussed above, a simple search of MEDLINE yielded over 1500 papers on CFS. The search only became manageable when the search was refined to randomised controlled trials that looked at treatment regimens. Consequently, to search Web databases effectively we need to construct the search question in a similar manner. Table 13.3 examines a number of search engines and gives examples of how searches can be refined.

### Search analysis

Both AltaVista and Northern Light returned an almost identical number of hits (18,801 and 18,868, respectively) when searching for the phrase 'chronic fatigue syndrome'. As the results from Northern Light are automatically arranged into discrete subject/domain folders – such as government sites, personal pages, etc. – refining any search is both easy and intuitive. In this example, selecting the folder 'government sites' reduced the number of hits to 301. At all levels, selecting more specific search folders can further refine the search.

**Table 13.3** Web search engines

---

**Google**             <http://www.google.com/>
Google is the biggest search engine on the Web, providing users with access to an index of more that 560 million pages. Moreover, because of the way Google uses link data, it can return listings for sites it has never visited, thus giving it coverage of just over 1 billion pages.
Unlike other search engines, Google returns a list of search results where the ranking is based on how other sites link to that site. So confident are the developers of Google of their search software that they invite users to select the 'I'm feeling lucky' button after a search term has been entered. On selecting this, users bypass the traditional search results page and instead are taken directly to the site Google ranks as being the most relevant to that search.

**AltaVista**             <http://www.altavista.com/>
Indexes 350 million pages. Use the 'refine' search option to select relevant topics and discard irrelevant ones. Use the 'advanced' search form to construct a query that uses Boolean operators. Also, use the special search syntax features that AltaVista supports. For example, to ensure that the phrase 'chronic fatigue syndrome' appeared in the title of a Web page, and that the page has a UK domain, the following Boolean search could be constructed: title:'chronic fatigue syndrome' AND domain:uk. Full details of all these search features can be found on the AltaVista Help page

**Northern Light**         <http://www.northernlight.com/>
Combining an index to around 265 million Web sites with its own special collection of full text journal and newspaper articles, Northern Light provides health professionals with a rich and, at times, unique source of information.
The Northern Light search engine sorts search results into discrete 'custom folders' which groups like-data together based on the subject, source of information (government, commercial, personal pages, *etc*.), language, and the type of information. Using the Power Search option you can restrict a search by source, language, date and the type of information. This latter filter allows you to specify variables such as events listing, learning material and company information (Fig. 13.3).

**Inference Find**         <http://www.infind.com/>
Inference Find is a meta-search tool that queries six search engines simultaneously and then merges the results, removes duplicates and clusters the results into understandable groupings. Although Boolean operators can be used, if Inference Find queries a search engine that does not support these operators then the results many not be as anticipated.

---

Google, as would be expected, yielded the biggest number of results – some 71,000 pages. However, the advanced search features are not as well developed as those employed at Northern Light and consequently refining this search is far more difficult. (Google is far more effective search tool when you are trying to identify the Web site of a known organisation.)

With Inference Find, all the search results are displayed on a single page and arranged by category headings such as 'chronic fatigue syndrome', 'miscellaneous European sites' and 'miscellaneous commercial sites'. The clustering of like-pages is a particularly useful feature and one which other Web search engines should adopt. For example, rather than point to all the relevant Web pages hosted by organisations such as the American Fibromyalgia Syndrome Association or the Chronic Syndrome Support Association (CSSA), Inference Find simply directs you to the appropriate home page.

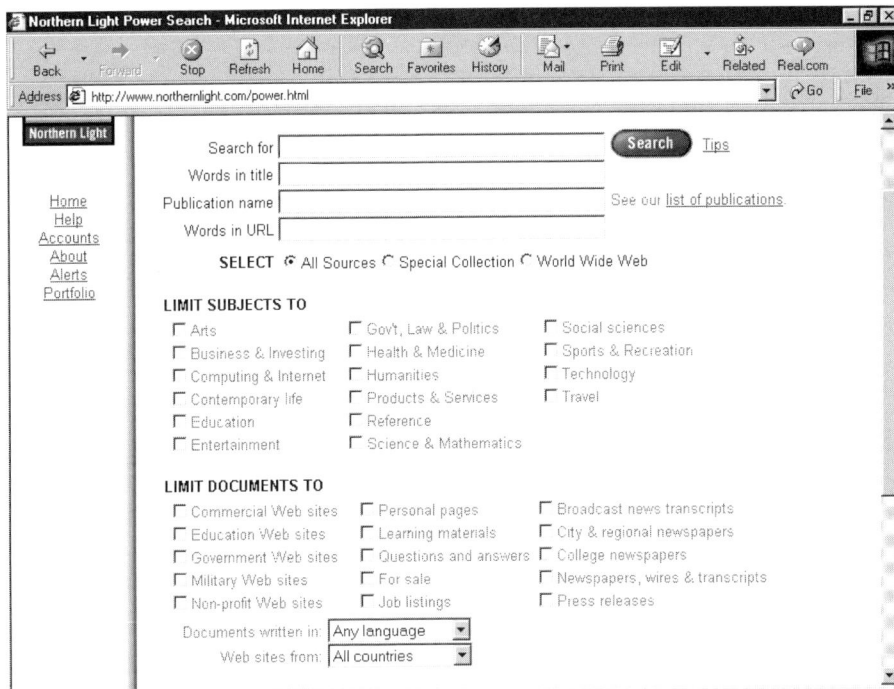

**Fig. 13.3** Sophisticated search options at Northern Light.

For more information about the various search engines, and tutorials on how to use these engines effectively, see <http://www.searchenginewatch.com/>

## Step 4 – Discussion lists and newsgroups

Internet discussions lists and newsgroups are another potential source of useful information. Although much of the debate in these forums may be anecdotal and lacking a research base, they do nevertheless provide an insight into the views and opinions of health consumers and professionals. For example, a student nurse who wanted an understanding of the distress experienced by chemotherapy patients would find newsgroups such as <news://alt.support.cancer/> and <news://sci.med.diseases.cancer/> most illuminating.

Identifying relevant newsgroups, and discussion lists can, however, be a time-consuming process. Indeed, current estimates suggest that there are approximately 80,000 newsgroups and 90,000 discussion lists catering for virtually every interest and speciality. Table 13.4 highlights the main Internet directories for identifying relevant newsgroups and discussion lists.

### Search analysis

Using the Interest Finder <http://www.deja.com/home_if.shtml> and entering 'chronic fatigue syndrome', DejaNews quickly identifies the newsgroups

**Table 13.4** Discussion lists and news groups

---

**DejaNews**    <http://www.deja.com/usenet>
DejaNews provides an on-line archive of all postings made to Internet news groups. Power searching enables you to filter a search by date, language and forum.

**Liszt**    <http://www.liszt.com/>
Liszt is a directory of Internet discussion groups. The directory can be both searched – by keyword – and browsed using broad Yahoo-type subject headings.

---

<news://alt.med.cfs/> and <news://alt.med.fibromyalgia/> as being the most relevant. Hypertext links enable you to browse the contents of these newsgroups. If you are concerned that relevant postings may appear in other groups, for example <news://sci.med.diseases/>, the entire DejaNews database can be searched. Using the Power Search option, searches can be filtered by date, language and forum.

Searching the Liszt database for CFS identifies a number of potentially relevant discussion lists, including CFS-L (a general discussion list) and CFS-Y, a list aimed at younger people who suffer with this condition. Crucially, the Listz database also provides additional information about each list, including how to subscribe, the purpose of the list, and whether the list is open or moderated.

## Step 5 – Keeping up-to-date

One of the most effective ways of keeping up-to-date with new research findings is to run a monthly-update search on the key bibliographic databases, identified above. In many cases, however, this will require you to revisit each database, re-key your search and restrict the results to articles that have been indexed within the past month. (PubMed MEDLINE, for example, has a 'limit to articles published in the last 30 days' option.) Alternatively, if you are prepared to pay, then companies such as OVID <http://www.ovid.com/> and Silver Platter <http://www.silverplatter.com/> will enable you to define a search that will be run

**Table 13.5** Keeping up-to-date

---

**WebMedLit**    <http://webmedlit.silverplatter.com/index.html>
Describing itself as a 'medical headline service', WebMedLit provides users with a one-stop-shop to 30 medical journals, including the *British Medical Journal, New England Journal of Medicine* and *Journal of the American Medical Association*. What differentiates WebMedLit from the countless other Web sites providing links to medical journals is its citation database. This database allows visitors to search the contents of these 30 journals from one source and then provides the hypertext link back to the article (or abstract) at the individual journal's Web site. As WebMedLit indexes journals within hours of publication, it is a good way of tracking the very latest research.

**Moreover**    <http://w.moreover.com>
Promoting itself as the 'world's largest collection of Webfeeds', Morover provides free access to over 1800 news' sources.

---

Guide to Healthcare Resources on the Internet

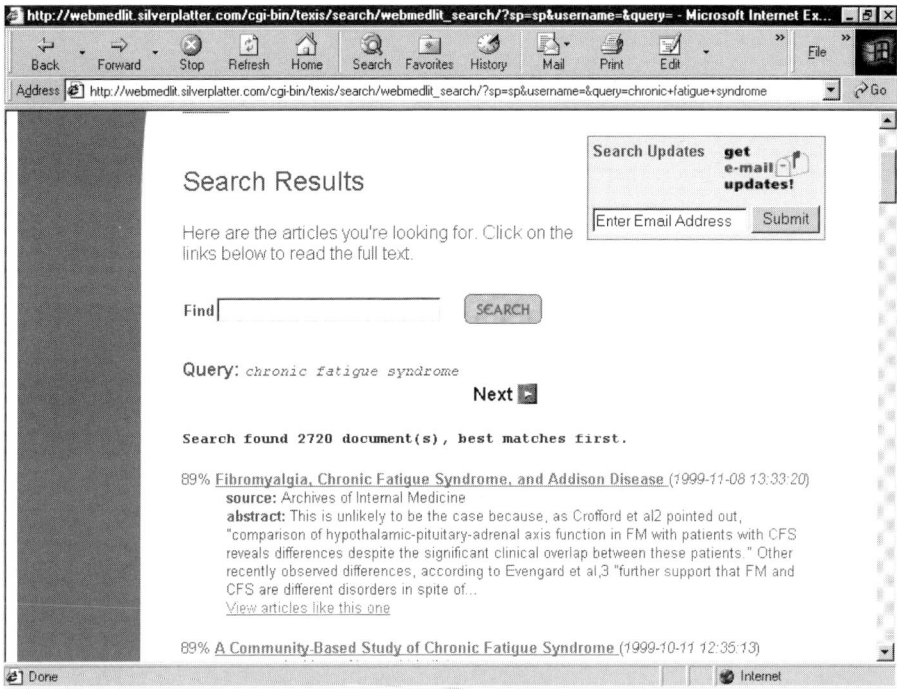

**Fig. 13.4** WebMedLit – a great tool for keeping up-to-date with current research.

automatically each time the database is up-dated. Any new citations that are retrieved are mailed to your electronic mailbox.

Table 13.5 details two other ways you can keep abreast of new stories and findings. Both these services are available without charge.

### Search analysis (Fig. 13.4)

Searching WebMedLit for articles on chronic fatigue syndrome identified a number of recent papers, including an article that examined the link between CFS and tobacco use published in the Archives of Internal Medicine[8]. In this example, the full-text of the article was available for viewing and printing free of charge. The WebMedLit service also allows you to bookmark your queries so you can re-run your query, without re-keying it.

Running a search on the Moreover service identified additional new stories including an article from a recent issue of the Independent newspaper ('Humans not designed for 24-hour living')[9] and a report that CFS was debated at the recent US Democratic convention. If a search identifies too many stories, Moreover allows the user to refine it by news source, topic or geographic location.

# Conclusions

Data from RelevantKnowledge – a leading provider of on-line marketing intelligence – shows that the most trafficked sites on the Internet are the Web-based search engines. Indeed, the 'Top 10' for August 2000 included six search engines[10]. Nowhere in this list is there mention of any of the online databases or evaluated gateways discussed in this column, despite the fact that a recent survey indicated that around 43% of US adult Internet users – 15.6 million people – go online to find health information[11]. The clear inference of this is that most Internet users are using the general Web search tools such as Yahoo! and AltaVista as a way of finding on-line health information.

This article has attempted to introduce a hierarchical approach to searching the Internet. At the top of the hierarchy are the databases that provide expert commentary on published research (Cochrane Library) and those, like MEDLINE and Embase, that index peer-reviewed research. If these sources do not answer your question then the next step is to search the evaluated subject gateways. In due course, further information can be found via general search tools and through on-line discussion forums. As you move down the hierarchy, however, it becomes increasingly important to evaluate the information that you find.

Although the quantity of information on the Internet is daunting, this article has demonstrated that relevant and timely information, from a huge variety of sources, can be found relatively easily.

## References

1  Chronic fatigue syndrome *BMJ* <URL:http://www.bmj.org/cgi/collection/chronic_fatigue_syndrome> [Accessed 28 August 2000]

2  CO-CURE. To subscribe send the message SUBSCRIBE CO-CURE YourFirstName YourLastName to: <listserv@listserv.nodak.edu>

3  CFS-DOC. To subscribe send the message SUB CFS-DOC YourFirstName YourLastName to: <listserv@list.nih.gov>

4  CDC <http://www.cdc.gov/ncidod/diseases/cfs/cfshome.htm> [Accessed 28 August 2000]

5  Chronic fatigue syndrome. Resources for patient. NIAID. <http://www.niaid.nih.gov/factsheets/cfsreso.htm> [Accessed 28 August 2000]

6  Web surpasses one billion documents <http://www.inktomi.com/new/press/billion.html> [Accessed 28 August 2000]

7  Search engine sizes <http://www.searchenginewatch.com/reports/sizes.html> [Accessed 28 August 2000]

8  Aaron LA, Buchwald D. Tobacco use and chronic fatigue syndrome, fibromyalgia, and temporomandibular disorder. *Arch Intern Med* 2000; 160(15): 2398–401. <http://archinte.ama-assn.org/issues/v160n15/full/ilt0814-8.html?3997e76082> [Accessed 28 August 2000]

9  Humans not designed for 24-hour living *Independent*, 1st June 2000 <http://www.independent.co.uk/news/UK/Science/2000-06/24hour010600.shtml> [Accessed 28 August 2000]

10  MMXI Europe – The Top Ten <http://www.mediametrix.com/data/thetop.jsp> [Accessed 28 August 2000]

11  Brown MS. Healthcare information seekers aren't typical Internet users. *Med Net* 1998; 2: 17–8

# Index